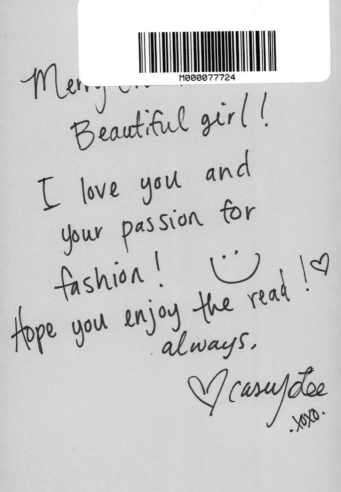

Mer~~~~ ~~~~~
Beautiful girl!
I love you and
your passion for
fashion! :)
Hope you enjoy the read! ♡
always.
♡ casy Lee
.xoxo.

THE
WELL-DRESSED LADY'S
POCKET GUIDE

KAREN HOMER

PRION

This edition published in 2016 by Prion
an imprint of Carlton Books Limited
20 Mortimer Street
London W1T 3JW

First published in 2012 by Prion

10 9 8 7 6 5 4 3 2 1

A CIP catalogue record for this book is available from the
British Library.

ISBN 978 1 85375 970 3

Senior Executive Editor: Lisa Dyer
Managing Art Director: Lucy Coley
Copy Editor: Jane Donovan
Design: Design to Print Solutions
Picture Research: Jenny Meredith
Production: Maria Petalidou

Printed in China

CONTENTS

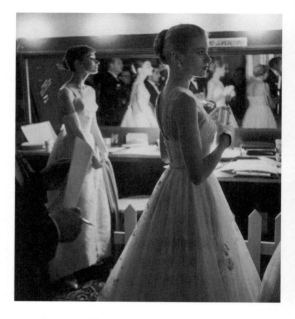

"*Dress shabbily and they remember the dress;
dress impeccably and they remember the
woman.*" Coco Chanel

INTRODUCTION

Women have always sought to be well dressed but what that means today is less clear than in previous times. In fact, from looking at photographs in gossip magazines or watching women on reality television shows, it might seem the art of dressing well is a dying one. Ill-fitting, poorly made clothes and choices inappropriate to the occasion are commonplace and a universal agreement on what is stylish has been replaced by the 'anything goes' school of dressing. Which makes it hard for the woman who wants to dress well, yet is unsure of quite how to go about it.

Luckily, there are still role models – both young and more mature – who manage to capture that combination of classically stylish, yet not out-dated. Think of the Duchess of Cambridge and her many sartorial triumphs or even her mother-in-law, the Duchess of Cornwall – another example of dressing appropriately for her age, her shape and the occasions she attends. And among the sea of celebrities on Oscar Night, there are always a few dresses that stand out from the garish and over-the-top concoctions worn by their contemporaries – usually simple, beautifully-cut, fitting like a glove and in keeping with the dignified mien of women such as Cate Blanchett and Nicole Kidman, modern style icons as Grace Kelly and Audrey Hepburn once were, half a century ago.

Historically, women have always looked to the higher ranks in society for guidance on what to wear. From the ancient world to the grand courts of Europe, it was usually royalty who set the trends, which then filtered down at least to the strata immediately below and often influenced the common woman as well. The full, long skirts of the eighteenth and nineteenth centuries, for example, were universal. And style etiquette such as always to wear a hat (and usually gloves, too) when leaving the house was observed by all until the 1940s; only beggars did not cover their heads.

It was in the first half of this century that style began to change but it was still the aristocracy who set trends, with up-and-coming debutantes gracing the covers of fashion magazines and filling the popular society pages of newspapers; women like Diana Mitford and later, Gloria Vanderbilt. And while the advent of the fashion designer might have given flamboyant individuals of humbler origins (iconic names, including Chanel herself, are famously self-made) more influence over trends, the wealthy and influential were for many years the public face of their collections.

With the disappearance of universal fashion etiquette and previously unimaginable social mobility over the last 50 years, it might seem the wish to be well dressed, with its connotations of snobbery and elitism, has fallen out of favour. But many women realize they want a style that endures – essentially classic, yet still individual, giving a nod to fashion but always appropriate. And while good clothes can be more expensive when compared to the disposable attitude to fashion – buy it cheap, then throw it away – compiling a well-thought-out wardrobe that will cover any occasion is more economical in the long run. And that's exactly what this pocket book for the well-dressed woman will teach you how to do.

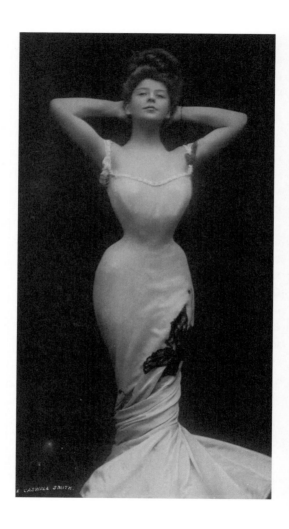

E CASWALL SMITH.

SHAPES AND SILHOUETTES

HISTORY OF THE FEMALE FORM

Women come in all shapes and sizes and while today's aesthetic might be for the elongated ultra-slim forms of fashion models, it has not always been the case that waif-like equals desirable. Aztec and Egyptian fertility goddesses had exaggerated shapes indicating a preference for high levels of body fat, and in the seventeenth century, Rubens famously popularized a voluptuous female form in his paintings. More recently, a smaller waist has become fashionable, but the androgynous shape we associate with beauty today was considered scrawny, unhealthy and even poverty-stricken until the 1960s. Compare, for example a picture of Marilyn Monroe to one of Keira Knightley – while both actresses are undeniably beautiful women, their body shapes are very different, illustrating the cliché that "beauty is in the eye of the beholder". Dressing well will allow any woman to look – and feel – beautiful.

BODY SHAPES AND DRESS SILHOUETTES

Whatever your shape, the key to looking well dressed is to dress appropriately to your figure. The female body can be roughly categorized into four shapes, though the difference within these is wide and not every woman fits completely into one or the other. Knowing what shape your body leans towards helps in choosing a dress silhouette that will flatter any figure.

PEAR OR TRIANGLE

This shape is often associated with the classic English figure. Narrow at the shoulders and often small-busted, the waist of a pear-shaped woman can be tiny, particularly in proportion to her hips and thighs. It is this waist/hip ratio that is often cited when it comes to studies determining a woman's attractiveness to men: the greater the difference between waist and hip, the more fertile (and therefore attractive to the opposite sex) a woman is supposed to be!

Yet finding clothes to fit is difficult in a world full of fashions designed for straight up-and-down figures. Choose clothes that accentuate the waist, such as bias-cut wraparound dresses or 1950s-style A-line

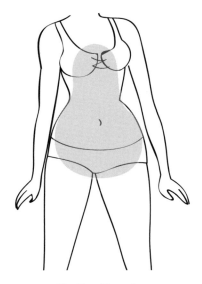

The Pear/Triangle

skirts with a fitted shirt tucked in, a neat sweater or a tailored jacket ending at the waist. Boot-cut trousers balance larger thighs and with heels, will elongate the leg and you can accentuate your waist with a belt. Wearing one colour (and yes, black is slimming) on top and bottom also helps minimize a difference in the size of both. Colour blocking, where you wear contrasting colours on top and bottom, only accentuates any difference in size. Avoid loose, baggy tops (sometimes chosen in an attempt to disguise a figure that a woman is unhappy with) at all costs: these will only make you look larger all over.

APPLE/INVERTED TRIANGLE

Opposite to the pear, the main difference is that the shoulders of an apple-shaped woman are broad compared to her narrower hips. Legs and thighs are slim and, in some cases, the upper body can look out of proportion to the lower half. These women are often conscious of carrying extra weight on their stomachs. Apples are not always overweight, however. The most obvious "inverted triangle" is the woman who appears "top-heavy" with an out-of-proportion bust, becoming more common with the popularity of breast enhancement operations – think Dolly Parton.

Perhaps surprisingly, wearing a bias-cut dress or top can work for these women, too – so long as it is not too closely fitted or in a very clingy fabric such as silk jersey. The idea is to minimize proportions and for a woman who feels she has "no waist", it can be enlightening to realize wearing clothes that accentuate the waist make one appear slimmer after all. The same applies to jackets and coats: choose one with a belt to exaggerate your waist.

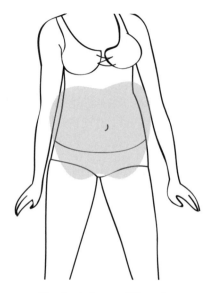

The Apple/Inverted Triangle

Knee-length shift dresses that gently tailor in towards the dress also emphasize a wider waist. As with the pear shape, a baggy top is tempting to conceal a large tummy, but be careful: many apples opt for skinny trousers over a very loose top but you may look out of proportion or even pregnant, particularly if you choose a flared or empire-line style! By all means opt for slim trousers, pencil or knee-length skirts (beware of skimpy minis) to show-off good legs but match them with a top that is neither too tight nor too baggy. A lower-cut T-shirt or camisole beneath a jacket or shirt can minimize a large bust and darker colours on top reduce large busts and wide shoulders. Avoid polo-necks, particularly if your bust is large and your shoulders are wide.

HOURGLASS

This figure is traditionally regarded as the perfect female shape, so go ahead and dress to accentuate your genetic good luck! Nevertheless, while the proportions of an hourglass are similar, the actual size of the individual woman will always vary. So, as with all body shapes, avoid covering up if you feel you are too curvy and instead choose relatively fitted classically cut clothes to emphasize your figure.

The ladylike fashions of the 1950s are ideally suited to this shape and fitted two-piece skirt suits or dresses in fine fabrics such as silk or viscose will all look excellent. Stiff fabrics are not such a good choice as they will fight your curves rather than flatter them. Similarly, ostentatious details such as ruffles or wild patterns, accessories like big belts or voluminous smock tops all kill the natural elegance of your figure, which needs no embellishment. Just remember, tailored clothes are your best friends.

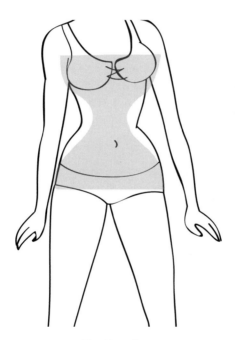

The Hourglass

RECTANGLE/BANANA

Not unlike the apple when it comes to advice on how to dress, this shape varies widely between the androgynous model with a distinct boyish lack of curves to the once-labelled "matronly" figure. Essentially, this definition applies when the bust and hip measurements are relatively equal and a woman has little in the way of a defined waist. Naturally, the slim, boyish model has few problems wearing any silhouette, but even she might wish to create a bust and waistline for herself by wearing tops with details such as ruffles that add fullness to the bust, perhaps tucked into a high-waisted skirt to accentuate any curves.

A larger rectangle should follow the advice for apples in accentuating the waist with belts and wrap dresses but, unlike the apple (who often has proportionally wide shoulders), a rectangle might choose jackets with shoulder pads and a tailored waist to achieve an elegant, shapely silhouette.

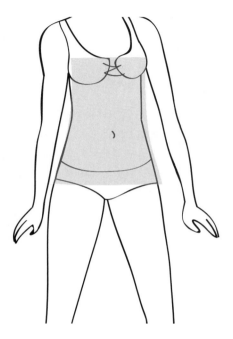

The Rectangle

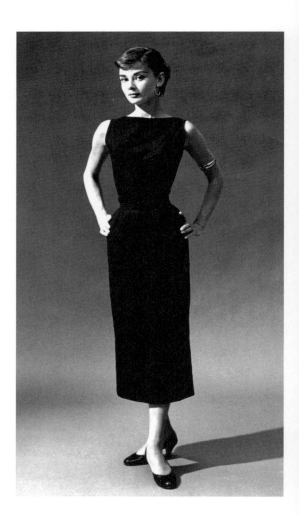

DRESSES

HISTORY OF THE DRESS

We take it for granted that we have many different styles of dress to choose from, though historically, dresses have been of one distinct style according to the era and society. For example, in ancient Rome, Greece and Egypt, dresses are well documented and similar for both men and women. They were made primarily from linen, occasionally dyed, but commonly left to bleach in the sun to a pristine white. Women's dresses were more modest than those of men, usually comprised of a simple sheath with shoulder straps, perhaps with the addition of a shawl or type of wrapped sari. Any expression of fashion or individuality was achieved by the addition of wigs or jewellery rather than different styles of clothing.

In the early Middle Ages, medieval women were still wearing simple sheath dresses or tunics, often capacious and sometimes with a cloak on top, but as the centuries progressed the distinctive medieval style of dress, featuring a tight bodice and voluminous skirt, began to emerge. Row upon row of impractical buttons, tight-fitting embroidered jackets bedecked with heavy jewels and long trains made these garments a real challenge to wear. The arrival of corsets – first worn over, then under tight bodices and padded rolls at the back of skirts – set the scene for the fashions of first the Tudors and later the styles of the seventeenth and eighteenth centuries, where women (albeit mainly those of high class) had to suffer arrangements of padded whalebone and steel to form the exaggerated wide panniers so popularized by Marie Antoinette.

The eighteenth century, with its fashion for a tightly corseted waist, exaggerated hips and a deep décolletage, is one of the first examples of how dresses were created to manipulate the female form to fit a perceived cultural ideal These extravagant gowns were in keeping with the sumptuous lifestyles led by many of the aristocrats, but the fashion filtered down to women of lower classes, who also favoured full skirts, nipped-in waists and a low-scooped neckline. It was not until the aftermath of the French Revolution when the aristocracy became so despised that looser, more informal styles of dress became fashionable.

Although in the first part of the nineteenth century a higher-waisted, looser dress was popular, it was not long before the tightly corseted waist became fashionable once more. By the 1850s, the hoop-underskirt (often made of thin wire) was popular and within a few decades, the bustle appeared, becoming bigger and bigger until the turn of the twentieth century, when it all but disappeared. The extremely tight corset also became less popular as women began to suffer health problems including digestive issues from a bound stomach and of course serious difficulties with childbirth. Nevertheless, this was an era when being fashionable became a popular preoccupation for many women and by the early part of the twentieth century, gossip about which dresses were in vogue had become a mainstream interest.

It was of course the First World War that liberated women from the structured dress. Clothes became more practical and showed the influence of military styles with braiding, belts and even boots for women similar to those worn by the soldiers. Postwar then, the rollercoaster of changing fashions really picked up speed. From the flapper dresses of the 1920s through the demure, chic and ladylike 1930s into the utilitarian styles of the Second World War and the celebratory, flamboyant New Look popularized by Christian Dior in the 1950s, women's dresses changed shape and length with the seasons and everyone watched and copied trends. Through the barely-there minidresses of the 1960s to the hippie tent-like creations of the 1970s, the changing shape of the dress throughout history is a veritable whirlwind of vastly differing styles. And that is why today, when fashion is so much about reinterpreting what has gone before, choosing the right dress can be a minefield. There is no one style that everyone who is fashionable is wearing; each season, designers give us a myriad of styles to choose from. That said, for the woman who always wants to be well dressed, there are certain templates to choose from, many of them harking back to the decades when ladylike chic was *de rigueur*.

THE DAY DRESS

Few garments are as useful to the well-dressed woman as the day dress. At its best a good dress is timeless, versatile, comfortable and flattering. On the flip side, of course, a bad dress may be more unforgiving than any other outfit. Choosing the right shape, skirt length, print and colour can prove daunting, particularly when confronted with such a wide spectrum of different styles, but the triumph of the dress is its versatility, so once you've got it right, there's no need to worry about finding a matching top, as with a skirt. Choose an appropriate weight of cloth for the season and a dress needs no jacket or cardigan to spoil the line, yet a good basic frock can be "dressed" up or down as the occasion demands.

DIFFERENT STYLES OF DRESS

When considering a style of dress, it is important to know which cuts suit your particular body shape and also, especially if you don't have unlimited space or a sky-high budget, which dress is the most versatile and can be adapted for different occasions. The dresses listed below are designed for daywear though some will work just as well for smarter occasions. For other dresses, such as cocktail dresses or ball gowns, please refer to the Eveningwear chapter (*see pages* 106–13).

SHIFT DRESS

The shift might well be seen as the modern equivalent of the everyday simple sheath gown worn by women in previous centuries and it is just as useful. First appearing in the collections of designers Hubert de Givenchy and Cristóbal Balenciaga in the mid-1950s, and popularized by style icons such as Audrey Hepburn and Jackie Kennedy, it epitomizes the ladylike chic so resonant of that era. Essentially similar in shape to the unstructured, sleeveless sheath of the 1920s flappers, this is a very different dress – less glitzy, more sober; better suited to the office, or to a simple lunch date than dancing Gatsby-style and champagne-fuelled into the early hours.

As such the shift is the staple dress of the well-dressed woman's wardrobe. Traditionally sleeveless and with a simple round neck, falling to the knee (or occasionally, slightly above or below), it has darts at the bust to give a neatly tailored and flattering shape and usually falls straight from the hips to knee-length. As with most dresses, fashion dictates subtle changes – an A-line or tulip skirt, or a capped sleeve would still allow a dress to qualify as a shift. Similarly, fabrics differ widely; the wool gabardine beloved of Givenchy and his contemporaries is certainly the shift's original cloth and undeniably elegant, but manmade fabrics or lightweight cotton can work just as well.

There are few body shapes that this style does not flatter if you follow some simple rules when choosing a shift. A small bust will benefit from a shift that fits closely at the waist, thus accentuating what is there; those with a larger top half should opt for a dress that skims rather than clings – as with all dresses, a well-fitting bra is essential. The fact that the shift is often in a block colour helps those who feel they are top or bottom heavy by creating a unified line. Women with narrow hips might choose a more tulip-shaped skirt; those with wider hips, a slightly flared or A-line shape. A more structured fabric such as Givenchy's trademark wool or heavy linen will alleviate the slightest body insecurities.

Lastly, the shift is the ultimate dress-it-up/dress-it-down garment. The ladylike cliché of pearls, pillbox hat, trim jacket and matching kitten heels and handbag so beloved of Grace Kelly and Jackie Kennedy in their public appearances might be slightly over-the-top nowadays but a short, gently tailored or classic boxy jacket will smarten up a shift while a neat cardigan will give a more vintage feel. Add knee-high boots and you will be channelling a 1960s vibe. A scarf instantly lifts a plain dress out of the ordinary, while a hat and brooch make it suitable for a wedding. Really, the possibilities are endless and a variety of shifts in different colours and fabrics are essential to the well-dressed woman's wardrobe.

SHIRTWAIST

If the shift is the modern equivalent of a workingwoman's everyday sheath, what is known variously as the shirtwaist or shirtdress became the twentieth century's answer to the frilly, ruffled blouse and long skirt of the Edwardian period. At this time the term "waist" referred to the bodice or blouse part of a woman's dress (ruffles and frills were as popular among men as women in those days). Many workingwomen in the late 1800s and beyond began choosing a more masculine blouse, both for comfort and as a sign of increasing independence – the style was popular with suffragettes, for example – but the style really exploded in popularity during the 1950s, giving us the iconic "shirtwaist". Initially, this was a neat shirt, teamed with a separate full skirt – think Audrey Hepburn as she stepped onto the silver screen in *Roman Holiday* (1953) wearing a simple blouse, full, belted skirt and neckerchief. It quickly evolved into a dress of one piece, where the top half was essentially a man's shirt complete with buttons and collar, complemented by a feminine full A-line skirt. Like the classic shift, this style of dress is inextricably linked to Fifties style but has evolved down the decades to become a simpler long, straight shirt, buttoned right to the hem and worn loose or belted. Today, it is more commonly known as a "shirtdress".

The shirtdress is a casual style, usually made of cotton, either plain or printed, and is a useful component of a Spring/Summer wardrobe. A relaxed and forgiving style to wear, it is suitable for all body shapes and far more flattering on a hot day than a skimpy, spaghetti-strapped minidress. The most elegant designs tend to hark back to the 1950s, with a blouson top and full skirt, sometimes with an attached fabric belt tying either at the front or back. Such a dress might have three-quarter length sleeves or sleeves that can be buttoned up; a sharper, more contemporary design could be a slim, tailored long shirtdress perhaps accessorized by a smart belt, making an essentially casual style of dress suitable for smarter occasions.

SWEATER DRESS

A slightly newer innovation and an obvious cold-weather equivalent of the shirtdress is the sweater dress. It is commonly thought to be a 1960s invention, popularized by designer Mary Quant, whose bottom-skimming dresses were barely longer than a normal sweater – think Jane Birkin in a somewhat see-through crocheted sweater dress on the arm of Serge Gainsbourg

– but the trend caught on and today sweater dresses are beloved of both designers and the high street.

The best of the sweater dresses tend to be a somewhat less structured version of the shift – and of course, with sleeves. Rather than choosing something that really does look like an oversized sweater – unflattering, whatever your size and shape – take advantage of the myriad of sweater dresses on the market. A simple knitted black sweater dress is a useful addition to a winter wardrobe but many designers tend to go to town with blocks of vibrant colour; stripes also work well.

The sweater dress is often made from a very fine jersey, which can be extremely elegant, or a fine merino wool or cashmere worthy of the wardrobes of the world's best dressed women. But while a dress can look wonderful when first worn (and the reason why women who possess mountains of beautiful cashmere always look fabulous is that they have enough sense *not* to over-use them!), these fabrics have a tendency to pill or the threads to pull out, or simply to go baggy. In fact the most beautiful designer sweater dresses would probably not stand up to everyday wear, unlike a hardy shift. That said, the appeal of the sweater dress is as a comfortable one-piece garment that may be smartened up with a jacket or coat or dressed down by wearing over trousers, jeans or leggings.

WRAPAROUND DRESS

The knitted jersey, wraparound dress is one of those unique shapes that suits wildly differing body types. It might seem like an obvious choice for the ultra-slim, with its essentially figure-hugging silhouette, and it does give the illusion of curves on a woman with a pencil-figure. Nevertheless, this garment also looks superb on a voluptuous woman; if you have a small waist and proportionally large bust and hips, it will accentuate your curves in a subtle way and even women who feel they cannot wear a wraparound dress because they have no waist to speak of will see one miraculously appear with a well-fitting dress.

It is impossible to think of the wrap dress without thinking of Diane von Furstenberg who, in the early 1970s, could be said to have invented it and has become synonymous with this design of dress. It helped that her socialite friends and impeccable connections embraced the new style so that it appeared everywhere in the

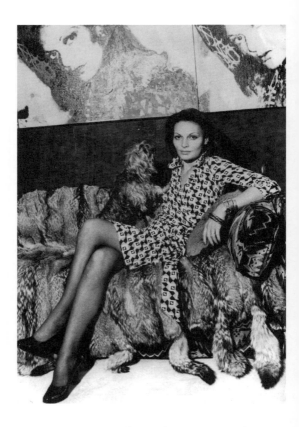

Diane von Furstenberg in her iconic wrap dress.

highest echelons of society and the photographs filtered down to a fashion-conscious public. Other designers and high-street stores were quick to jump on the bandwagon of this easy-to-sell style. In fact, the wrap has become so iconic in its influence on women's fashion that a fine example features in the Costume Institute of New York's Metropolitan Museum of Art.

One final reason why the wraparound dress should be included in the wardrobe of the well-dressed woman is that it suits all age groups. Young women can easily carry off the often-flamboyant prints and colours but the style and vibrancy is also a good alternative to the sometimes staid dresses aimed at older women and will make an impact, whether worn in the office or to a more formal occasion.

MINIS, MIDI AND MAXIDRESSES

Before closing this chapter, it is worth talking a bit here about the fashion for different dress lengths. When designers first started showing the new season's collections it was all about the hemline – was it up or down? Today there is such a wide variety of designs shown that what is in vogue is not quite so clear-cut but there are certainly seasons when the mini- or the maxidress is back in, as well as the recent popularity of the more demure knee-length or mid-calf ladylike styles beloved of designers such as Miuccia Prada. If you have the confidence, the legs and the lifestyle, by all means wear a minidress – after all, French women insist a short skirt and a pair of heels are key to their enviable style. Similarly with maxidresses, if you are tall, slim and on vacation somewhere that socialites gather, a wildly printed, tanned-shoulder-bearing maxidress will look stunning. But exercise good judgement and bear in mind that most women who wish to appear classically well-dressed and want their newly purchased dress to last more than one season would do well to stick to lengths anywhere from just above to slightly below the knee.

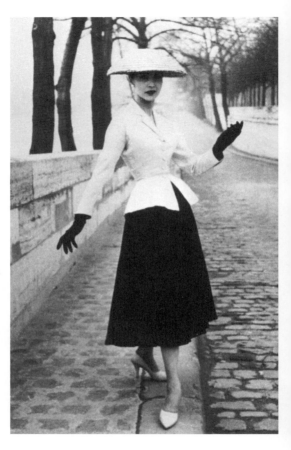

The Christian Dior "New Look" silhouette.

SKIRTS

For every woman who adores a dress, there are plenty who prefer the flexibility of a skirt and top – if only to limit their washing loads and dry cleaning bills! In fact skirts pre-date dresses as women's garments and have not dipped in popularity over thousands of years. And despite the gradual relaxing of dress etiquette over the last 100 years, which has allowed women the flexibility to wear trousers, the skirt is here to stay and is a stalwart of the well-dressed woman's wardrobe.

A BRIEF HISTORY OF THE SKIRT

Skirts have been worn by women (and men, too) for thousands of years – in fact, a type of skirt fashioned from string is one of the earliest documented forms of textile clothing, with examples dating back as far as 3,000 BC. Almost certainly, they were worn for thousands of years before this, as carved figures of women dating from as long ago as 20,000 BC include decorative string skirts, often as simple as a kind of apron at the front. These first examples of clothing are similar to the grass skirts that are still traditional costume in parts of the world such as Hawaii.

Although initially a simple adornment, skirts quickly became a source of both warmth and modesty associated primarily with women, with a few notable exceptions such as the Scottish kilt. For centuries, modesty demanded women's skirts were worn long and voluminous skirts were also seen as a mark of prestige – up until the Industrial Revolution, fabric was expensive.

Throughout the eighteenth century skirts formed part of a lady's gown, sewn onto a bodice and open at the front to reveal copious underskirts or "petticoats" (not the same as the petticoats of later fashions, which were undergarments only). Structured hoops, made of wood, metal or whalebone, were worn to give the skirt volume: in the sixteenth century this was known as a farthingale; in the eighteenth century the exaggeratedly wide pannier came into fashion, while the crinoline was essential to give structure to ladies' dresses in the nineteenth century. Similarly, bustles, bumrolls and rump pads were used to help support a skirt's frame, giving the skirts and gowns of these eras their characteristic accentuated rear.

Throughout the nineteenth century, skirts gradually slimmed down to become more streamlined and by the First World War, hemlines began to rise as a practicality due to the increasing number of women taking on war work. Throughout the flapper era of the 1920s, hemlines rose to around the knee in the characteristic beaded dresses but dropped again by the 1930s. The Second World War in the 1940s saw hemlines rise again, thanks to rationing of fabric, and despite still being in force after the end of the war in 1947, Christian Dior launched his iconic New Look, where he defiantly used 20 yards of extravagant fabric to create his signature full, mid-calf skirts with their many petticoats, incredibly (certainly to our modern figures) tiny waists and an accentuated bust. With women's sexual liberation in the 1960s, teeny-tiny miniskirts were in vogue but by the 1970s, a different take on Women's Lib led to long hippie dresses coming into vogue. And of course in the 1980s – the decade fashion prefers to forget – women endured the wide-shouldered, sharp-suited "power dressing" silhouette, with a short pencil skirt.

It is interesting to note how much skirt lengths have been affected by social and political change over the years, but in these days of endless sartorial freedom hemlines are rarely linked to economic crises. There are few situations in which a woman is expected to wear a skirt, although this is not unheard of, and the myriad of designs and styles available means the well-dressed woman can choose according to her own personal style rather than follow the vagaries of fashion.

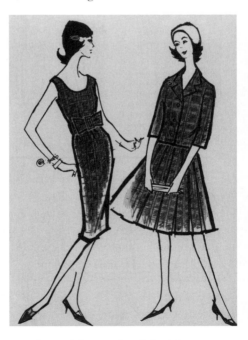

Two classics: The pencil and the A-line, c. 1957.

CLASSIC SKIRT SHAPES

Below is an overview of different skirt shapes befitting the well-dressed woman. These are classic looks that have worked for decades and continue to form the staple shapes in a modern-day well-dressed woman's wardrobe.

PENCIL SKIRT

This elegant, tailored skirt-shape falling from waist to knee is the essential skirt for anyone aspiring to be well dressed. Neatly fitting, it epitomizes the genteel chic of the 1950s, yet rarely has it fallen out of favour since then, although hemlines may dip just below or rise slightly above the knee, depending on fashion. The pencil skirt usually has a slit at the back but its close-fitting, somewhat unforgiving shape means it is best suited to immaculately slim figures.

For the ultimate 1950s look, the pencil skirt is teamed with a neatly fitting sweater or even twinset, pearls optional. But any tailored blouse or top will suit a pencil skirt for a stylish working outfit. A straight skirt (see below) is an acceptable alternative if you find a pencil skirt too figure-hugging. Accessorize with a slim belt, either worn on the skirt or over a sweater or cardigan.

STRAIGHT SKIRT

While lacking the simple elegance of the pencil skirt, a straight skirt – where waist and hem are approximately the same width – is a good alternative for those less confident about their figures. This shape is flattering to almost all body types and if you choose a smart fabric such as wool gaberdine rather than a denim or heavy cotton, it can be teamed with much the same tops as a pencil skirt.

A-LINE

With its neat waist and flared shape, the flared A-line skirt is the diametric opposite to the fitted, slim pencil. It is nevertheless classically elegant and favoured by many of the style icons from the 1950s and 1960s who also wore pencil skirts – for example, Jackie Kennedy. This shape is an ideal alternative to a pencil skirt for those with larger hips and can be worn with exactly the same type of neat sweater, blouse or cardigan.

A-line skirts are ideal for summer as they are best made from attractive, lightweight fabric such as cotton lawn. Printed skirts, particularly in the slightly vintage prints and colours that have become so popular with designers in recent years, should be a summer staple.

CIRCLE SKIRT

Not dissimilar to the A-line, the circle skirt is essentially named after the hemline, which forms a perfect circle. Rather than giving the accentuated triangle and flare of an A-line skirt, the circle is full and works similarly well in lightweight printed fabrics for summer. It can be less flattering to those with larger bottom halves than the A-line, though, as it is fuller at the waist and does not flatten across the stomach in the same way.

MINISKIRT

The miniskirt is cautiously included in the list of appropriate skirts for the well-dressed woman simply because of the chic Frenchwoman's love affair with a short skirt. There are stylish short skirts and inappropriate ones, though. If you are lucky enough to have the legs to carry it off, by all means wear a neutral, one-colour, subdued, short (but not *too* short) straight skirt. And don't go for overkill by revealing cleavage at the same time: subtlety is the essence of the Parisian style, which the well-dressed woman would do well to emulate. No matter how perfect your figure, rather than squeeze into a rear-skimming, leopard-print mini, choose a short skirt, classic heels and an elegant blouse or jacket instead.

SKIRT SHAPES TO AVOID

TULIP SKIRT
The tulip skirt is shaped exactly as it sounds – an upturned tulip head – and it is virtually impossible to carry off unless you are a catwalk model. Even then, although it is arguably fashion-forward, it is not "well dressed".

BUBBLE SKIRT
Not dissimilar to, but far worse than the tulip, the bubble is best left to small girls off to fifth birthday parties or game-for-a-laugh women prepared to sacrifice style for a 1980s costume party.

GYPSY SKIRT
While not always unattractive, the flared, almost flamenco-style gypsy skirt has such a 1970s feel that it is impossible to recommend this style for the woman who wishes to be classically well dressed. If you are after the kind of bohemian rock-chick look that is admittedly carried off by celebrities such as Sienna Miller (or has certainly been so in the past when the look was in vogue), the gypsy skirt, in its trademark printed fabrics, is spot-on. However, if you aspire instead to a subtler expression of elegance, steer clear of the long, full gypsy skirt!

MAXISKIRT

Sometimes similar to the long gypsy skirt, the maxi is a usually less flared and can even resemble a garment once worn by a Victorian schoolmistress. This is a hard look to pull off and while fashion-focused celebrities barely out of their teens might attract the style paparazzi by wearing one, most other women should avoid them. Apart from anything else they are hopelessly impractical as you are almost always treading on the backs of your hem.

MERMAID/FISHTAIL

The mermaid skirt (and similarly the mermaid dress) is tight to the hips and thighs, then flares out showily in a fishtail from the knee to the floor. In fact this style was so beloved of the glamorous icons of the silver screen, such as Marilyn Monroe and Jayne Russell, it could qualify for the well-dressed woman's wardrobe.

However, being pure 1950s high-octane glamour, the fishtail skirt or dress demands a similarly starry occasion (think Oscar Night), few of which the average modern woman has call to attend. It is also an overtly sexy style of dress – the fishtail tends to complement a daringly revealing top half – which goes against the well-dressed woman's essentially discreet style.

BLOUSES
AND SHIRTS

One of the easiest ways to appear well dressed as opposed to shabby is by wearing an elegant blouse or crisp shirt with your chosen skirt or trousers. The word "blouse" might conjure up dated images of a pussy-bow-wearing, handbag-toting Margaret Thatcher, but the blouse has experienced something of a revival in recent years and is favoured by many leading designers for a truly ladylike look. And similarly, there are few pieces as fresh and sharp-looking as a masculine-style shirt, but the two looks are very different so it is worth mastering when to choose blouses and when to opt for shirts, and learning which suits your individual shape and style the best.

HISTORY OF THE BLOUSE

For many centuries, the blouse was associated with peasant garb and therefore too informal for the smartly dressed woman as there were few situations where such loose, unstructured garments could appropriately be worn. By the

Edwardian 1890s, however, the practicality of the blouse, plus the need for somewhat less formal clothes as women entered the workforce in greater numbers, saw a leap in popularity. And by the early part of the twentieth century, women who worked in offices and as schoolteachers and governesses made the blouse and long skirt their uniform of choice: smart, yet comfortable. At this time blouses were made of cotton or silk, depending on the status of the woman, and did not always include a collar.

While working women might choose a demure blouse, in the early part of the last century many blouses were more elaborate. One particular style was named the "lingerie blouse" as it was decorated with the type of lace and embroidery more suited to underwear. And the "Gibson Girl" blouse was named after the popular female ideal created by illustrator Charles Dana Gibson at the end of the nineteenth and the beginning of the twentieth century. With her slender, yet voluptuous hourglass figure, this icon of beauty remained popular for several decades and the blouse was similarly shapely, with tucks and pleats that emphasized the bust and nipped it in at the waist. It became immensely popular for both informal occasions and even some eveningwear.

In fact, more modern interpretations of the Gibson Girl blouse are still popular today.

This tailored style of blouse emphasizing the female form continued in popularity and introduced a garment that was very different from the peasant garb or artists' smocks formerly associated with the term. Seams and darts at the waist, though used even in Victoria times, became more accentuated by the 1930s, thus bringing the blouse into the realm of smart daywear. Variously made from silk, cotton lawn or linen, the blouse was neat fitting, with small buttons and tailored sleeves. By the 1960s, and with the advent of manmade fabrics, viscose and polyester became popular, easy-care alternatives although the true well-dressed woman should note crackling nylon is not the most elegant choice.

It is hard to exactly distinguish the blouse from the shirt, particularly when blouses were plain and made of cotton with simple pointed collars, but there are a few examples in the 1950s of distinctively masculine-style shirts such as the cowboy-style checked shirts Marilyn Monroe was photographed in, daringly paired with blue jeans. However, the decade when the shirt really came to the fore was the 1980s, when the trend for masculine dressing meant that blouses looked outdated; instead crisp, sharp shirts better suited the similarly angular business suits that were in vogue.

The gentlemen's tailors of Savile Row traditionally supplied customer's shirts along with their suits and as demand gradually increased, these tailors began designing both shirts and bespoke suits for female clients. True men's shirts have a double cuff for cufflinks and are longer at the back, with a tail to tuck into trousers. The double cuff is perhaps not necessary for a woman's shirt but many designers (and female customers) like this feature. Fashion designers who have latched onto the superior tailoring of men's clothes – for example, British designer Margaret Howell, who made her name selling the perfect crisp white shirt – still make shirts for women that are longer at the back. Of course these shirts are also tailored to accommodate a woman's bust and waist.

Perhaps the most obvious difference between men's and women's blouses and shirts is that men's buttons are on the right, women's on the left. The historical reasons for this are unclear but traditionally, men most often drew their sword from the left hip with their right hand. To avoid the risk of a sword catching a button, they were therefore sewn onto the right side. In the seventeenth century, when only the wealthy could afford buttons and women were dressed by maids, it was easier to do so with the buttons on the left. Whether or not this is historically accurate, the tradition has stuck and women's buttons are always on the left.

COLLAR STYLES

For blouses and shirts, collar styles vary. Many of the differences are subtle but it is worth illustrating the most common ones.

PETER PAN COLLAR

Small, softly rounded collar found on many blouses. Has a slightly vintage feel about it.

POINT COLLAR

As the name suggests, these collars have a slightly pointed edge and can be worn laid out flat or turned to stand up in the style so beloved of Princess Diana in the 1980s. On a very masculine shirt or a woman's dress shirt, the point collar is sometimes exaggerated.

BUTTON-DOWN COLLAR

Similar to the point collar, only with a button

to keep it down and help the shirt collar remain impeccably crisp.

CHELSEA COLLAR
This collar is designed for a shirt or blouse with a deep V-neck (for example, a sleeveless summer shirt), with long points; it was popular in the 1960s and 1970s.

JOHNNY COLLAR
A slightly shallower V-neck collar for open-neck blouses.

JABOT COLLAR
This is a simple collar with a ruffled or pleated detail down the front of the blouse.

SHAWL COLLAR
A rounded collar to suit an open, V-neck blouse that is similar in shape to the neat Peter Pan collar, but larger and wider. Hence being named after a "shawl".

Peter Pan

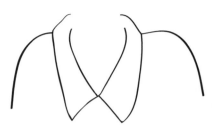

Chelsea

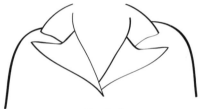

Notched

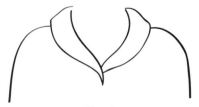

Shawl

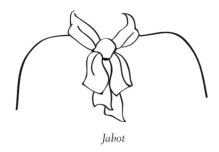

Jabot

ESSENTIAL BLOUSES

For anyone aspiring to elegance, a blouse is a key wardrobe addition. A simple white or cream silk blouse does not date, will suit pencil skirts or tailored trousers and adds a touch of femininity to a business suit. Coloured loose-fitting silk or cotton blouses are a beautiful counterpoint to more casual trousers – either cropped Capri-style or wide-legged in the original androgynous fashion of Coco Chanel in the 1920s. Blouses have become so beloved of fashion designers that there is a multitude to choose from: chiffon or silk-crepe are classic choices and come in a wealth of colours and delicate prints. Style icons such as fashion maven Anna Wintour are often seen in the trademark printed silk, somewhat vintage-feel blouses from design houses like Prada.

For a more streetwise elegance, take a leaf out of
the Parisian's style notebook and wear with slim
trousers or even smart dark denim, skinny jeans.
A loose top balances a tightly fitting bottom and
the juxtaposition of fabrics gives a thoroughly
modern chic that our Edwardian ancestors could
not have imagined.

A shirt is often interchangeable with a blouse
(sometimes it's hard to know why one garment is
labelled a blouse and another a shirt) and which
one you choose greatly depends on your own
personal style and shape. Those who like the
flirty and feminine blouse may also appreciate
its slightly more forgiving nature. The lighter
fabrics and lack of emphasis on darts and tailoring
minimize a larger bust, particularly if you choose
a detail such as a pussy-bow that draws attention
away from the chest. Shirts tend to be leaner and
suit, appropriately, a more androgynous figure.

The best shirt styles for simple elegance are
still feminine with a nod to androgyny and
their masculine heritage. Smart, plain-coloured,
with perhaps a subtle herringbone check, truly
tailored Savile Row-style shirts are a wardrobe
staple when you are expected to wear suits to
work. If the line still seems too sharp, soften

with a modern printed scarf from somewhere like Missoni rather than the somewhat staid traditionalists' Hermès silk square.

For a more relaxed style, there has been a renaissance in the checks and plaids reminiscent of the starlet beach-shots of the 1950s, which can still form part of a well-dressed woman's wardrobe if carefully paired with slim, dark jeans, tailored khaki trousers and perhaps tucked in with a neat belt to accentuate the waist. Even a simple pale blue chambray skirt worn with a matching A-line skirt and a tan belt would work.

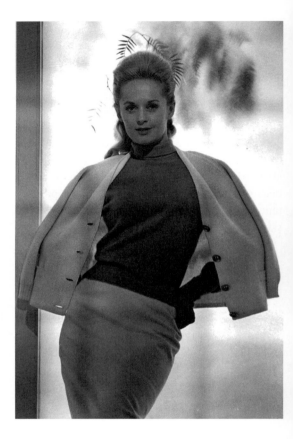

Tippi Hedren in a knit polo-neck and lined cardigan.

KNITWEAR

Certain garments are quintessentially ladylike – the silk blouse discussed in the previous chapter being one of them, beautifully simple knitwear another. There are many kinds of knitwear that belong in the well-dressed woman's wardrobe including 1950s-style neat twinsets, elegant, slim cashmere polo-necks and gamine, lightweight jersey Breton tops. All of these and more are essential pieces to combine with different styles of skirt and trousers.

A HISTORY OF KNITWEAR

Knitted fabric has been around for millennia. London's Victoria and Albert Museum features a pair of knitted socks excavated in Egypt at the end of the nineteenth century and dated circa the third century ad, although the technique used was more akin to knotting than the needle-knitting of today. Knitting, as we now know it, dates back to eleventh-century Egypt, when cotton and silk were knitted into socks and other garments. This was the first evidence of knitting using a two-needle technique; previously a single short needle was used to produce a crochet-like fabric.

The art of knitting was also popular in the thirteenth and fourteenth centuries in Europe – the Madonna is even depicted knitting in paintings of the time. Knitting guilds were formed with formal apprenticeship schemes that made the fabric more attractive to the wealthier classes; garments, including shirts, jackets and also stockings (worn by men too, of course) and lingerie were made from knitted silk fabrics, which had the advantage of being extremely stretchy. The most wealthy clients commissioned garments knitted from fine silver and gilt threads.

Wool only became popular as the skill of knitting filtered down to ordinary working people when practical, heavy fisherman's sweaters, warm shawls and babies' clothes were made. The Industrial Revolution saw knitting transfer from a small cottage industry into large-scale production, yet at the same time it became popular once again as a genteel hobby. Victorian women of status were expected to knit, and patterns began to be published and passed around for the first time. By the twentieth century and during the First and Second World Wars, women were required to "Knit for Victory", picking up their needles to help the war effort by knitting for soldiers. Items included socks, sweaters, helmet liners, scarves, caps and blankets. Everyone, from the ordinary woman to the British Queen and First Lady Eleanor Roosevelt, played their part in knitting to support the war effort.

Knitting continued to evolve throughout the twentieth century, with new techniques such as cabling appearing from Ireland in the early part of the century. From being the fashionable pastime of Victorian and Edwardian ladies, knitting has remained popular with film stars like Joan Crawford glamorizing the art in the 1930s and 1940s. Although with greater numbers of women putting their careers first in the latter part of the twentieth century when a domestic hobby like knitting might have been expected to fall from favour, it has experienced a renaissance of late with glamorous fashion editors seen pulling needles and balls of the finest wool from their designer handbags as they wait for notoriously late-running catwalk shows to begin. And movie stars such as Sarah Jessica Parker and Julia Roberts also confess to a love of knitting.

From a fashion point of view, the turning point came with Coco Chanel's innovative use of jersey in her iconic suits. The Chanel suit perhaps epitomized the liberation of women in that era and even today the knitted skirts and jackets are instantly recognizable. The sweaters and cardigans most often created from knitted fabric were also a mainstay of Chanel and other early designer's collections. Jean Patou, the designer most famous for his iconic scent "Joy" in the 1920s, created wonderful block-coloured knitwear inspired by the Cubist painters and he popularized cardigans as a fashionable but more natural and comfortable garment for his rich American socialite clients. The trend caught on and from the 1930s onwards, elegant knitwear has been a favourite of some of the most stylish women in history, including Jackie Kennedy, Audrey Hepburn, Grace Kelly and Elizabeth Taylor.

TYPES OF KNITWEAR

TWINSET
The iconic combination of a neat, often short- or cap-sleeved knitted sweater and matching cardigan is most evocative of the 1950s and '60s when popularized by film stars, including Marilyn Monroe and Audrey Hepburn. Worn with a pencil skirt and heels, or slim 1950s-style tailored, cropped trousers, it epitomizes casual elegance. While a twinset is sometimes associated

with frumpy older women in ill-fitting tweed skirts or with the upper-class cliché of "twinset and pearls", today it has become popular with fashion designers and young style icons who enjoy the retro, vintage feel. It is also an extremely practical, comfortable yet still smart alternative to the business suit, as originally worn in the 1950s and 1960s when popularized by working women such as secretaries (think Christina Hendricks playing Joan Harris in the hit TV series *Mad Men*).

The classic twinset is comprised of a closely fitting sweater that falls no further than the top of the hip and a round-necked cardigan of a similar length. Cashmere and fine merino wool are common fabrics although synthetic fabrics became popular in the 1960s. Usually a plain colour, pastels and pale neutral hues are most redolent of vintage chic but twinsets, particularly in cashmere, have become so popular that specialist companies will create the same pattern in a rainbow of shades. Variations on the theme include a sleeveless sweater and cardigan.

POLO-NECK AND TURTLENECK
The distinction between a polo-neck and turtleneck is slightly arbitrary but a polo-neck is often higher and sometimes worn flush against

the neck, although it can be folded down, whereas a turtleneck is either a single layer or a shorter, folded neck. These terms are generally interchangeable and refer to a high-necked sweater that rose in popularity in the mid-twentieth century, both with men as a smart alternative to a shirt and tie, and for women – in America, in particular – where it became the neat and tidy poster-sweater of the preppy student with A-line skirt and swinging ponytail. Like the twinset, it was taken up by Hollywood stars though worn in very different ways – the voluptuous Jayne Mansfield favoured a super-clingy, figure-accentuating polo-neck while the gamine Audrey Hepburn would pair a loose polo-neck sweater with slim trousers and ballet flats. The latter is probably more appropriate for the well-dressed woman, who tends to favour understated elegance.

There are many other contemporary ways to wear the turtle or polo-neck – in fact it is one of the most versatile additions to your wardrobe. A fitted, fine-knit, high-neck sweater will pair with tailored trousers (slim or wide-leg) and similarly smarten up dark denim. Skirts of most kinds can take a polo-neck, although the pencil skirt is perhaps your best choice. For a more modern look, a longer, looser smart cashmere polo-neck also works on a pencil skirt, particularly when teamed with beautiful, statement boots. On the whole, fine knits work better for ladylike dressing than chunky ones and super-fine polo-necks, perhaps with short or three-quarter length sleeves, make the style suitable for spring and summer. A word of caution for those with large busts, however: a polo-neck is perhaps not the best choice for you. While certain Hollywood starlets might have chosen the style precisely because it accentuated their assets, you may not wish to do the same.

ROUND-NECK SWEATER

A catch-all term for a variety of neat-to-the-neck sweaters, this is an incredibly versatile knit that will take a print or pattern better than a polo-neck. That said, the most elegant tend to be plain or simply striped and reasonably fitted. The "sloppy-joe" sweater, baggy and ill-fitting, as well as too casual to be elegant, has no place in the well-dressed lady's closet. A plain round-neck style also works well worn over a crisp white shirt or simple blouse and suits all body shapes.

V-NECK

This can be a delightful addition to a Spring/Summer wardrobe, particularly in lighter colours. Designers tend to favour deep V-necks and show them worn alone, but some women are less comfortable with a revealed décolletage so bear in mind that V-necks also suit being worn over a shirt or blouse. They are more flattering than a polo-neck when worn beneath a smart jacket and perhaps accessorized with a contemporary statement necklace. This is a good style for minimizing a large bust.

STRIPED, BRETON-STYLE PULLOVER

Although technically not a shape, this sweater deserves a mention of its own because it is so classically stylish. Since the 1920s, when Coco Chanel was daringly pictured in a boat-neck, striped Breton jersey belted into high-waisted, super-wide legged masculine trousers and tennis shoes, it has become an iconic top. Beloved of women everywhere, including Claudia Schiffer, Elle Macpherson and Alexa Chung, it is versatile, flattering and always chic. Worn with slim, cropped Capri pants, a 1950s-style A-line skirt, jeans or even shorts, it has the kind of relaxed style about it that the well-dressed woman needs for dress-down days and holidays.

FINE, MEDIUM OR HEAVY KNIT?

On the whole the most elegant knitwear is fine or medium in weight. Whether it is made from cashmere, wool, a silk-blend or a modern fabric-like modal, it will suit tailored bottoms – skirts, trousers or even jeans – better than a chunky knit. If you are conscious of any lumps or bumps, avoid super-fine knitwear, particularly in modern fabrics or silk jersey that tends to cling and can also be see-through. Instead choose a well-fitted cashmere or merino wool. And note lambswool can be extremely itchy so you may need to wear something underneath which might make it too chunky (or hot!). However, there are a few exceptions to the smooth-knit rule – for example, delicate cable-knitted sweaters.

EMBELLISHED KNITS

In recent years, designers have become extremely fond of embellished knitwear. Everything from lacy corsages to slogans, panels of glittery stripes to a pair of large sequinned lips bang in the middle of the chest has strutted down the catwalk but exercise caution: anything so overtly "fashion" is likely to contradict innate good style, plus it is a piece that will rarely last more than a season. Nevertheless, for eveningwear, a subtle sparkly or tastefully embroidered piece of knitwear may be seen as the modern equivalent of a lady wearing a flamboyant brooch. Discretion is still the watchword.

CARDIGANS AND CARDIGAN COATS

Classic round- or V-neck cardigans are very useful. The original layering piece (worth remembering in fickle climates), they can be worn over a simple jersey top, a blouse or shirt or even as a top in their own right, buttoned almost to the neck. As with other knitwear, choose a plain design and colour, as well as the highest-quality fabric (in general, choose natural over manmade), which will stand you in good stead.

The cardigan coat or jacket is a relatively new innovation that has become very popular. Although a long, unstructured cardigan might seem a little casual, there are many beautifully crafted pieces around that make a well-dressed alternative to a stiffly tailored jacket for many occasions.

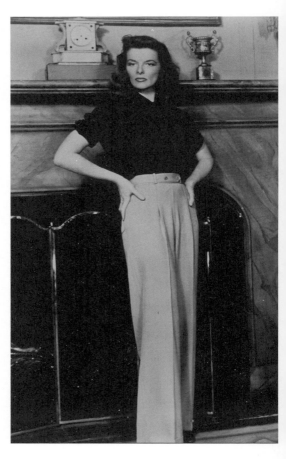

Katharine Hepburn in mannish tailored trousers.

TROUSERS

A HISTORY OF WOMEN WEARING TROUSERS

The modern woman takes it for granted that she can choose to wear a dress or skirt, as her ancestors did, or instead wear a pair of trousers appropriately tailored to the female form. If heads turn as she walks down the street, she can hope this is in admiration rather than shock, but it was not always so.

For centuries, women exclusively wore dresses or skirts. The concept of females wearing trousers was practically unheard of, judged to be anything from unladylike or undignified to downright scandalous. But in the nineteenth century, women involved in industrial work shocked prudish society when they began to wear trousers – for example, those working alongside their husbands in northern England coal mines needed more practical clothing and so they wore trousers beneath their skirts, which were then hitched high to the waist as they shovelled piles of coal. In the American West, women working on ranches also wore trousers throughout the nineteenth century. In fact, trousers as riding garb were one of the earliest acceptable forms of trouser for females.

In the 1930s, trousers began to be popularized by actresses such as Katharine Hepburn, Lauren Bacall and Marlene Dietrich, as well as by fashion designers including Coco Chanel, who borrowed shooting trousers from her lover, the Duke of Westminster, and let the tweedy dress codes of the English upper classes influence her designs for women. By the Second World War, partly as a result of clothes rationing but also for practical reasons as females took on much of the absent male workforce's jobs, women first began to wear their husbands' civilian clothes and then, as they acquired a taste for wearing trousers, they began to buy their own.

Nevertheless, despite the rise in popularity, trousers were still regarded as only suitable for manual work, chores like gardening, or leisure activities such as visiting the beach. Style icon Chanel was only photographed wearing long, wide trousers and a classic striped Breton top while visiting the French Riviera, otherwise she sported her trademark suits or skirts with blouses and knitwear. In the 1950s, the return to femininity and nostalgia for traditional homemaking that followed the end of conflict meant trousers were once again frowned upon, although actresses including Audrey Hepburn and Brigitte Bardot popularized the newly fashionable, slim, cropped Capri pants – Hepburn both off-screen and in movies, among them *Sabrina* and *Funny Face*.

The notion of women wearing trousers in a smarter environment was still much frowned upon in the 1950s, however, as is illustrated by the experience of Katharine Hepburn who, when visiting her beau, Spencer Tracy, at Claridges Hotel in London, was asked to refrain from wearing her trademark trousers in the lobby. She subsequently refused, instead preferring to keep her look and use the tradesman's entrance to the hotel. By the 1960s, however, trousers had begun to hit the mainstream and became more acceptable in all situations. In 1966, Yves Saint Laurent designed the iconic "Le Smoking" tuxedo dress suit for women, which became a classic that never dates. A decade earlier, the idea of wearing trousers in church would have been unthinkable.

The 1970s heralded a gradual acceptance of trousers for women in the workplace, but only among a few forward-thinking companies and only then, smart trouser suits. Iconic films such as *Annie Hall*, and the memorable trouser-wearing character played by Diane Keaton, helped to popularize the trend. Despite the vogue for masculine dressing in the 1980s, with a *Dynasty*-style silhouette emphasizing wide shoulders and slim hips, along with the appearance of trouser suits on the high street, it took several more years for certain professions, including courts and government offices, to condone trouser-wearing for women. Today it is deemed acceptable to wear smart trousers in almost all situations, while trousers as casual-wear are ubiquitous and, in fact, more common than skirts among younger generations.

TROUSER STYLES

WIDE LEG

For decades after women began wearing trousers the only choice was wide-legged. The earliest trousers in the 1930s, for example, were virtually indistinguishable from actual men's trousers (or, in fact, *were* men's trousers as Coco Chanel showed when she sported country-tweed plus-fours belonging to her beau). The style was exaggeratedly loose and long, with creased-fronts and pulled high to the waist, sometimes accessorized with a belt. Today's tailored wide-leg pants are not dissimilar to the original 1930s template that Chanel designed but they have been refined to avoid the unflattering "bunching" that would occur if one were to wear actual men's trousers. By all means choose pleat-fronted trousers as part of a suit but make sure there is no excess fabric around the waist. A side-fastening pair are often more flattering than a front-zip.

Chanel's "beach-style" of super-wide legged, flat-fronted trousers is still a winner and extremely elegant when worn with a striped sweater or a simple blouse, or even a plain, well-cut vest-top as the designer herself did on vacation. Heavy linen or cotton and dramatic (albeit impractical) white "sailor" trousers are an undoubted classic. Similarly useful in the well-dressed woman's wardrobe is the silk evening trouser. Worn with a blouse or an embellished top of some kind and strappy heels, this is an elegant look.

Many designers include wide-legged trousers in their collections when fashion nods its head back towards the 1970s, but this often means flared bottoms. Unless you have the panache and presence of the likes of Bianca Jagger or the long legs of Jerry Hall, this is difficult to carry off and also a style that quickly dates.

Wide-leg trousers suit slim women but also those who feel conscious of a large middle as the width will balance out apple shapes. If you are looking to project extra height, they are also a good bet as you can wear them draped to the floor over heels and high at the waist, giving the illusion of endless legs.

STRAIGHT LEG

The description "straight-leg trousers" is something of a catchall covering everything from classic tailored suit trousers to harem pants and drawstring trousers. Needless to say, the well-dressed lady should choose the first of these. Wool-twill or cotton (according to season), plain coloured straight-leg trousers are a wardrobe staple and perfect for teaming with blouses, shirts, sweaters, jackets or coats of all descriptions. By building up from a neutral palette of black, navy and beige and adding coloured or statement printed tops, this is an easy way to put together a stylish look. Best of all, the understated shape of straight-leg trousers is universally flattering.

NARROW LEG (AND LEGGINGS)

The vogue for narrow-leg trousers shows no signs of abating. Since Kate Moss made the skinny jean and trouser her trademark look when everyone else was still wedded to the bootcut, figure-hugging trousers and leggings have become ubiquitous. And despite appearing to be the preserve of the young and beautiful, there is a place for this style in the well-dressed lady's wardrobe. But integrating a more fashion-forward look must be done with care: choose high-quality fabrics – thick jersey, heavy stretch cotton or tailored wool-twill – and simple block colours. For an off-duty look, these trousers are the best choice for tucking into high leather boots, perhaps teamed with a simple polo-neck. If you have the panache to carry it off, a pair of high heels and a tailored jacket work equally well with narrow trousers for smarter occasions.

CROPPED/CAPRI
Not all cropped trousers are Capris but these slim, fitted and cropped-to-mid-calf trousers (originally designed with a small split and slight kick out at the bottom) are certainly the most stylish. Invented in 1948 by the European designer Sonja de Lennart, the original Capri pants were part of a whole "Capri" collection, so-named by the designer after her love of the island. Quickly taken up by holidaying socialites and actresses including Grace Kelly, Audrey Hepburn and Brigitte Bardot, and brought to public attention when worn by Mary

Tyler Moore in *The Dick Van Dyke Show,* they became instantly popular and have remained a classically stylish look.

Capri pants suit many tops – in particular, striped Breton-style boatnecks, as well as shirts, blouses and even neat T-shirts. Given their fashionable sun-soaked island heritage, they are one of the few styles of trouser that you can pull off in bright colours. For a vintage feel, pastels or brights work equally well when worn with a simple, crisp white shirt. More recently, the inherent classic chic of the Capri pant has been compromised as designers have produced leather and shiny Lurex versions and overly casual combat-trouser styles. Needless to say, sticking to the simple original is the best choice if you wish to remain well dressed. Wear with flat sandals, loafers or driving shoes or even plain, white retro tennis shoes.

JEANS

A HISTORY OF JEANS

Despite being probably the most ubiquitous form of dress in the West (and increasingly in many other parts of the world, too), denim jeans as we know them have been in existence for less than 150 years. First recorded as all-purpose trousers for the sailors from Genoa in sixteenth-century Italy (hence the root of the word "jeans" from the French *bleu de Gênes* or "blue of Genoa" and also the word "denim", as the first denim came from Nîmes or "de Nîmes"), the invention of blue jeans as we know them has been attributed to Levi Strauss in the 1850s. Strauss sold his eponymous blue jeans to the mining communities of California and in 1873, he invested in the idea of one of his customers – Jacob Davis – that copper rivets be used to reinforce points of strain on the trousers (for example, the pocket corners and base of the fly). A patent was granted and the all-American jean as we recognize it today was born.

Up until the Second World War jeans were worn only by labourers needing the resilience of the reinforced trouser, although both male and female workers in the factories during the war wore jeans: men's with a zip at the front, women's at the side. These loose "waist overalls", as Strauss originally dubbed them, were rather like a pair of overalls without the bib and a far cry from the fashionable close-fitting garments often seen today.

In the 1950s, American denim was adopted as the uniform of choice by cowboys and was regularly seen in movies starring the likes of John Wayne and Clint Eastwood, but jeans hit the fashion mainstream when James Dean wore them in the 1955 film *Rebel Without a Cause* and instantly created a style icon that became an essential part of being cool for a whole generation of teenagers. And for women, Marilyn Monroe set a new look in movies such as *The Misfits* (1961), though she also favoured denim in her personal wardrobe. There were plenty of less likely celebrities who adopted denim as their fabric of choice – for example, Bing Crosby, who from the mid-1930s onwards performed in his beloved Levis (the company custom-made denim Tuxedos for the star). As legend goes, he was once denied a hotel room, thanks to his attire – until being recognized, that is!

By the 1960s, jeans were becoming more common-place and women's jeans were now made with a central rather than a side zip; the Teddy-boy cult was borne from British rock'n'roll and along with it came the second-skin, otherwise known as the "drainpipe" jean. By the 1970s, jeans had been adopted as standard casual-wear, with different fits becoming more widely available and the first "pre-shrunk" versions patented by Hal Burgess. This was also the decade that saw the arrival of flared jeans: super-tight at the top and exaggeratedly flared at the bottom, ideally worn with super-high platform shoes.

In not much of an improvement, the 1980s marked the arrival of stonewash denim and a trend for denim jackets and shirts, ending with a revival of drainpipes that continued into the early 1990s. A dress-down aesthetic dominated the 1990s overall, which meant that jeans (along with trainers) were considered *de rigueur* for off-duty dressing and denim began to be accepted more widely, even in some trendier working environments. Towards the end of the 1990s, Alexander McQueen introduced the super low-waisted jean and gave women something new to worry about as tops were suddenly too short to cover stomachs – something young, toned and often tanned women took full advantage of. Bellybuttons appeared, uncovered, up and down the high street.

Since the turn of the century, jean styles come and go. For many years, bootcut was the style of choice, but more recently skinnier jeans are back in vogue. Even flares have seen a revival, albeit in a less exaggerated form than the original 1970s incarnation. Denim has darkened to a deep indigo over the years, too, which is good for those who wish to look smart – if not for their light-coloured upholstery. Today's well-dressed woman has an almost endless choice in what fit, style and colour of jean she wishes to wear and there are few occasions now where denim is unwelcome. Getting the right fit is a matter of trial and error, though, and the difference in styles is subtle, but there are some pointers listed below.

JEAN STYLE

STRAIGHT LEG

If you are looking for one pair of jeans to keep in your wardrobe, the straight-leg, mid-rise dark denim is the one to choose. As it sounds, this is a fit flattering to almost every figure other than the very pear-shaped and it can look extremely elegant worn with a simple white shirt tucked in, or a plain knit topped by a tailored jacket or classic trench coat. A fantastic all-rounder, the bottoms of a pair of straight-cut jeans are narrow enough not to look baggy when tucked into boots but also wide enough to accommodate heels or flats.

SKINNY LEG

Similar to the straight leg but obviously somewhat narrower in fit, the skinny leg has become the uniform of choice for models and celebrities, probably because it helps to be equally skinny in order to pull this style off. Nevertheless if you do have a perfect figure to emphasize then a dark, understated pair of skinny jeans can be worn in the same way as straight legs. A word of caution on jean-leggings (or "jeggings" as they have been dubbed): while you might think this is a comfortable alternative to getting the skinny-jean look, it is almost always possible to tell the difference between legging-jeans and true skinny jeans as the former are usually made of an inferior cotton. If you are prepared to pay a small fortune for a pair of designer denim leggings and have the figure of a supermodel, choose the darkest pair with appropriate fake jean pockets and you might just get away with it.

WIDE LEG

Overall, a more casual look and one with a distinctive 1970s vibe, wide-legged jeans differ from flared in that they are wide all the way down. This is a harder style to pull off, but one of the nicest ways is to choose white, lightweight wide-leg jeans for a summer look, perhaps teamed with tan platform sandals and a bright sweater.

FLARED

Again, a more casual look and similar to the wide-legged jeans described above, although some pairs will be narrower at the thigh and then flare out more obviously at the calf. These also work well for a Spring/Summer look, in a lighter, more washed denim to suit the more casual style, with sandals and a colourful top or even a printed blouse. This is a more fashion-forward look than a wardrobe staple, such as a classic pair of dark jeans.

BOOTCUT

This is still the style considered by many women to be their safety net. Tight on the hip and thigh, then falling straight to the calf, where the jean then flares out slightly, it is literally named because you can fit a boot beneath the legs. For years this was the standard style of jean and it is still the best choice for women of a certain age or those with wide hips because the flare at the bottom will balance them out. The joy of the bootcut is that it can be worn with boots underneath but also with heels or flats and is unlikely to fall out of fashion. Like the other classics, these jeans work best with simple shirts or blouses and a jacket if your aim is well-dressed elegance. For an injection of Parisian chic, a more playful, feminine blouse (perhaps in a pastel colour or print, but still with elegant sandals) is a nice way to feminize a pair of jeans.

HIGH-, MID- AND LOW-RISE

The waists of jeans have fallen as low as barely above the panty-line and also gone as high as a woman's true waist, but the more versatile rise is the mid-rise, reaching above the hips but nowhere near your true waist (the narrowest part of the torso). These jeans don't risk a bulge of stomach (or "muffin top", as it has unattractively been named) and are suitable for tucking in shirts or wearing with all but the most cropped of tops. Low-rise jeans are still popular with many women, partly because of the individual shape. Some short-bodied females might find a low-rise more comfortable and similarly those who are short in the crotch may find high-rises cut in. For those with an impeccable figure and washboard stomach, the low-rise feels much the same as the mid-rise, though there is always the risk of revealing a "builder's crack" when bending forward – possibly one of the most unappealing sights of all! High-rise jeans are sometimes chosen to cover bulging stomachs (older women often fall into this trap), but covering a potbelly with denim may feel reassuring but actually look terrible because it exaggerates rather than conceals the problem. High-rise jeans can also dig in uncomfortably when you sit down. Again, perfect figures can take their pick of styles but if you have any imperfections (and who doesn't?), mid-rise is your safest bet.

WASHES

Dark, dark and dark is the mantra if you want your jeans to have a truly stylish look. A uniform indigo wash is smart enough to team with high heels and an evening top and jacket, or wear to work with a tailored jacket and shirt. For more casual styles, however, there is no reason not to choose a lighter wash – particularly good when paired with bright summer colours and tan sandals. White jeans, despite the slightly 1980s association, actually look great for chic holiday wear. Avoid at all costs acid-washes, printed jeans, embellished jeans, or designer "ripped" jeans if your intention is to always appear well dressed.

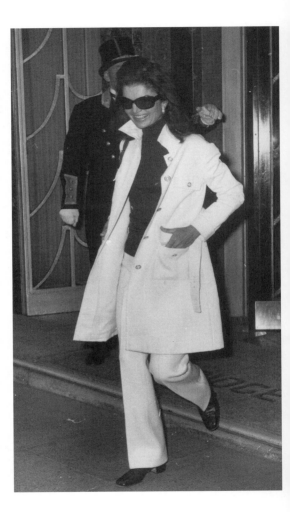

COATS AND JACKETS

A BRIEF HISTORY

The term "coat" is one of the earliest documented references to clothing, dating back to the Middle Ages. Originally used to refer to chainmail (as in "coat of mail") and variously spelt "cote" as well as today's "coat", the term quickly came to mean a fitted, buttoned outer-garment. The word "jacket" comes from the Middle-French word *jaquet*, meaning a small or lightweight tunic. "Coat" and "jacket" are often used interchangeably in modern speech (particularly in American English), while coat is also used in reference to particular forms of dress such as the gentleman's "tailcoat".

In the nineteenth century, when copious layers of dress were commonplace, a distinction was made between over-coats and under-coats; the most helpful way today of distinguishing between a coat and a jacket is to equate the "overcoat" of the past with today's "coat" and the "undercoat" with a jacket (the former being long; the latter, short).

For example, both men and women might wear a tailored blazer-style jacket beneath a waterproof or warm wool overcoat depending on the season. There was even a trend, back in the 1980s and 90s, to wear a denim jacket beneath an oversized, long, wool coat.

Part of the reason why historically coats were more often associated with the gentleman's wardrobe is that until the late nineteenth century women's gowns were so voluminous that they preferred a cape or shawl to a coat, which would have been impossible to fit over the top. A short, fitted jacket was the most a nineteenth-century female might have worn. By the end of the century, however, as day dresses slimmed down, coats became fashionable for women and were designed for a number of pursuits, particularly sporting pursuits such as hunting. Coats were needed for other practical reasons, too – for example, the trend for bicycling and then motoring meant outer garments were required to provide protection against wind, dust and rain. The earliest motoring coats were high-collared, long, double-breasted and heavy to survive the inevitably uncomfortable journey in early motorcars, becoming lighter as automobile comfort improved. In the early part of the twentieth century ladies' coats were elegant as well as practical, drawing on traditional masculine designs for inspiration – for example, the fashionable velvet-collared Chesterfield coat, double-breasted, tailored to the waist and flaring to a finish at the hip, and the similarly tailored but ankle-length female version of the travelling coat.

Shortly before the outbreak of the First World War, and with the Women's Suffrage Movement gaining ground, fashion began to turn away from corsets (*see also pages* 137–9) and tight-fitting long dresses for females. In their place softer, draped lines and a trend for bold prints from the Orient became popular. But the need for women to take up war work meant a complete departure from both the new fashions and the former rigid Edwardian dress strictures. Uniforms, including trousers, were commonplace for women as well as men, while coats and jackets adopted a similarly military feel with tunic-jackets, belts and epaulets. Perhaps the most important coat to be popularized as a result of the war was the trench coat, so-named for its all-purpose usefulness, in the trenches and beyond.

Originally developed as an alternative to the heavy (and fatally water-absorbent) serge great coats favoured by British and French soldiers, British firm Aquascutum lays claim to a trench coat design dating back to the 1850s but in 1879, Thomas Burberry developed a new, lightweight, weather-proof fabric known as "gabardine". In 1901, the company submitted a design for an army officer's coat to the British War Office. While never compulsory and only permitted to be worn by the highest rank of serving officer, who had to purchase them privately, the trench coat had arrived and its popularity remains undiminished. During the Second World War many countries adopted a version as a practical part of a soldier's uniform but more importantly, the trench coat became fashionable for civilians and is one of the first notably masculine styles to be adopted by women. Immortalized by actresses such as Ingrid Bergman in *Casablanca* and Audrey Hepburn in *Breakfast at Tiffany's* and hugely popular among stylish women off-screen, too, few coats epitomize chic as well as the trench.

Typically for times of peace after a war, both the 1930s and 1950s saw a return to feminine chic, which for women's coat and jacket fashions meant elegant, flowing evening coats and short, neat, tailored jackets with matching long, slim dresses – for example, the Schiaparelli designs so beloved of Wallis Simpson. Masculine influence never quite disappeared though, as Schiaparelli, along with Coco Chanel, enjoyed experimenting with tailoring – using severely padded shoulders – long before the 1980s.

Fur coats, despite controversy towards the end of the twentieth century, were also ubiquitous in its first half, particularly among the aristocracy as an indicator of wealth and status; also for their practical warmth. By the 1960s, coats had simply begun to follow the fashion of the day: mid-length, colourful and reasonably unstructured, often with a fur collar to be worn over minidresses. Fitted tailored jackets were also in vogue – again worn with short skirts as part of a suit, with matching pillbox hat, bag and shoes, as favoured by Jackie Kennedy. The trend for matching coats and dresses continued into the 1970s but fell out of fashion in the 1980s, with the new masculine power dressing. During these decades and beyond, coats and jackets have become fashionable in every fabric imaginable: leather, denim, fake fur, rubberized cotton – even the Mary Quant plastic poncho-style cape became iconic.

Today's well-dressed woman is spoilt for choice when it comes to coats and jackets. Nevertheless, there are certain types of coat that are essential components of a stylish wardrobe.

BASIC TYPES

TRENCH COAT

The trench is an essential part of the well-dressed woman's wardrobe. Adored by style icons as diverse as Jackie Kennedy and Kate Moss, there is barely a fashionable woman who does not wear one regularly. It is the most versatile of coats, smartening up casual jeans and tops but also equally well suited to a dress. The basic mid-length trench in a neutral colour is an obvious choice, but short, cropped versions, voluminous longer ones and those in brighter colours can work well. Best of all, it suits every body shape.

PEA COAT

Similar to the military-style coat in its uniform feel, the pea coat was originally worn by sailors. Double-breasted, it reaches the hip and sometimes has brass buttons. The lapels are often wide and the waist nipped in, making this coat a stylish daytime choice, as demonstrated by Jackie Kennedy. America's former First Lady was such a fan that the style is sometimes known as the "Jackie O".

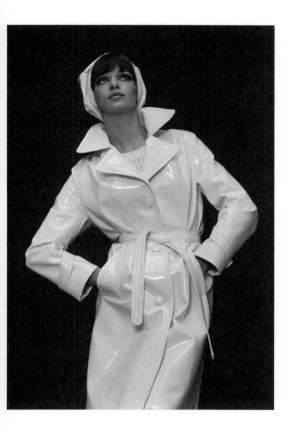

WOOL OVERCOATS

There are many styles of heavy woollen overcoat, depending on your style and personal preference, most being modified versions of traditional male coats – for example, the single-breasted Crombie is a subtly tailored mid-length coat, useful for wearing over suits or, if you prefer, the double-breasted Chesterfield is similarly straight, with just a little definition at the waist. Both are good basic winter coats, particularly if you choose a top-quality wool or cashmere in black, navy or camel.

The belted, wrap-coat is another example of a classic wool coat, with more femininity and elegance about it than the styles described above. With no buttons and fabric that wraps over at the front to be tied with a belt, it is elegant and versatile. Again, choose neutral colours and top-quality fabric.

Similar to the trench in style, the military coat is obviously made from a heavier fabric, either wool or a synthetic, and hardwearing. The key details are that the coat is double-breasted, usually long and has a belt. It often features brass button detailing or epaulettes.

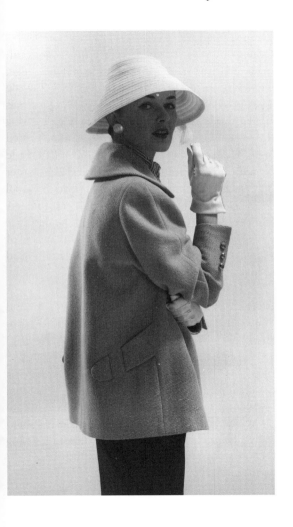

DUFFLE COAT

Originally made of a thick, coarse fabric from the town of Duffel in Belgium (from whence it takes its name), the duffle is also a traditionally English style of coat, thanks to the company Gloverall standardizing the duffle look in the 1950s when they began using buffalo horn toggles with leather fastenings and their trademark checked fabric. As with other traditional coats, the duffle has a military heritage, this time with the British Navy. There is a place for a duffle in the well-dressed lady's wardrobe – and not necessarily only for the young – but be sure it is top-quality and also traditional as it is a distinctive look and more casual than any other woollen coat.

PARKA

The parka is the ultimate casual cold-weather coat but very difficult to describe as elegant. That said, if your lifestyle demands practicality, there are stylish, well-made, neutrally coloured versions that look good with jeans and have a certain streetwise chic about them. Warm, waterproof and generally useful for inclement weather, the parka has been made fashionable as "festival chic" wear by models such as Kate Moss.

SHEARLING

Over the last few decades, the shearling has risen in popularity as a super-warm alternative to a woollen coat. Despite the vast cost of these garments, with designer versions running into thousands of pounds, there is a danger of looking overdone when wearing a shearling coat, particularly the floor-length, "hairy" versions. A neat shearling jacket can be a stylish choice, especially when worn with an elegant pencil skirt and heels.

LEATHER COATS AND JACKETS

Similar to shearling, leather needs to be very well thought out in order to look stylish and not suffer a clichéd "footballers' wives" fashion overkill. A simple, buttersoft tailored leather jacket or mid-length coat will suit some women, perhaps teamed with a pencil skirt, tailored trousers or even as a striking textural contrast to a pretty dress. Be careful to avoid full-on, overly embellished biker-style jackets.

BLAZERS OR TAILORED JACKETS

Incredibly useful items, blazers or tailored jackets have witnessed a real renaissance of late, with designers such as Stella McCartney making them something of a trademark. Worn over skirts or tailored trousers or used to dress up smart jeans with heels, a good blazer is a staple of the well-dressed woman's wardrobe.

DENIM JACKETS
It is hard to see how these could be included in the elegant, well-dressed woman's wardrobe, given their essentially casual nature. However, if you are a fan of denim, there are occasional exceptions – for example, the dark denim blazer.

CAPE JACKETS
A recent trend has been for the cape jacket, which actually harks back to those early motoring coats. This can look great if you choose carefully, although they are not the most practical of garments as your arms are never properly covered and on some women, they can appear too bulky.

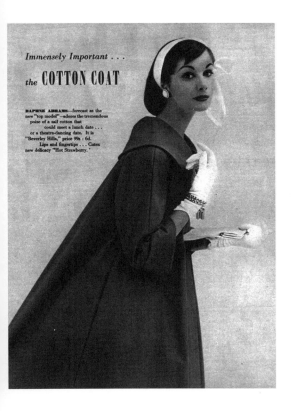

Immensely Important . . .

the COTTON COAT

DAPHNE ABRAMS—forecast as the
new "top model"—adores the tremendous
poise of a sail cotton that
      could meet a lunch date . . .
or a theatre-dancing date. It in
"Beverley Hills," price 99s : 6d.
    Lips and fingertips . . . Cutex
new delicacy "Hot Strawberry."

OFFICEWEAR

A BRIEF HISTORY

Until the last century women rarely worked outside the home unless they were in domestic service and uniformed accordingly. Single women in the nineteenth century were employed as governesses and teachers, wearing the fashions of the day for long, reasonably practical skirts and high-necked blouses, but it was not until the late-nineteenth century that females began taking on clerical positions. In the early twentieth century women's suffrage and the liberation offered by the First World War allowed women to replace men in many areas of civilian life, meaning more females held office positions for which they dressed practically and sensibly in line with wartime austerity.

By the 1930s secretarial schools were springing up and produced a battalion of elegant and identikit women, dressed in neat suits with white gloves, matching hats, shoes and handbags, ready to enter the typing pool. With clothes rationing in force during the Second World War and beyond, fashion became more sombre during the 1940s, but women still wore skirts, jackets, blouses, hats and gloves daily as a matter of course. In the 1950s, however, peacetime saw the arrival of Christian Dior's "New Look" celebrating the glory of femininity, and working women revelled in showing off full skirts with layers of petticoat, tiny nipped-in waists, long gloves and high heels; hats were still worn. Not everyone embraced the trend, though. In fact, 700 female office workers in Louisville in the USA signed a petition against the New Look.

It is impossible to talk about 1960s office styles without conjuring up images of the cult television series *Mad Men* and advertising agency staff dressed in neat dresses, pastel cardigans and pearls. The fashion from the series may be a little hammed up, but in the early 1960s, it was still *de rigueur* for working women to wear shift dresses, little heels, cardigans or jackets and to accessorize with pearls and often gloves and a hat, too. Jackie Kennedy might have been on official state business as opposed to working in the secretarial pool but the fashions were not so different. Skirt lengths rose in line with trends as the decade progressed and the cliché of a male boss dressed in a smart suit and his clutch of female support staff in pretty dresses remained.

Despite a second wave of women's liberation in the 1970s and feminists such as Gloria Steinem urging women to refuse to learn typing as a protest against the subjugation of females, more and more of them were entering the workforce. Skirts were still the norm and fashion trends had the biggest influence on working women's choices: miniskirts were still popular, as were dresses. In the 1970s, these changed from pretty pastels to crackly synthetic fabrics boasting bold geometric prints and bright colours; from the mid-1970s, muddy shades of green, brown and rust featured. The characteristic 1970s shirt with its exaggerated lapels was loyally worn by many women throughout the decade, including First Lady Pat Nixon, but the fashion for either hippie maxidresses or flared trouser suits is unlikely to have had much of a presence in the workplace despite popularity elsewhere. However, 1972 did see Diane von Furstenberg create the jersey wrap dress that has become a modern staple for women, both in and out of the office (*see also* *pages* 29–30).

Think of workplace fashion in the 1980s and "power dressing" is what immediately springs to mind. Though not universal, it was certainly a trend among more senior women, who wanted to emphasize that they were just as capable and influential as men – their chosen battledress being the *Dynasty*-style suit with shoulders padded to the max à la Joan Collins. Trouser suits also started to appear, although in contrast to the heavy shoes of the 1970s, there was a return to the pointed, kitten-heeled styles of the 1950s. Even women who chose to wear the silk suits and dresses that were fashionable in the 1980s bought into the trend for exaggerated shoulder pads that were virtually ubiquitous, even appearing under sweaters.

Since the 1990s, the dress code for women in the workplace has gradually relaxed; 1980s suits faded into a generally softer aesthetic, with tailored skirts or trousers and smart separates deemed perfectly acceptable. The biggest change in officewear over the last 20 years is the advent of casual dress for the workplace, first in media companies such asmagazine publishing or advertising agencies and later in New Media start-ups, where it is usual to see the entire workforce, from CEO down to work-experience trainee, dressed in jeans and trainers (albeit designer brands).

WHAT TO WEAR TODAY?

These days, workplace dress guidelines are often ambiguous, to say the least. When building a working "uniform", it is essential to take into consideration the nature of your profession and to take your cues from what other women (particularly your boss) are wearing. If you work in a profession such as law or another corporate environment, the dress code will inevitably be stricter than in a media company, where skinny jeans might be totally acceptable.

Suits are still a safe bet, as are tailored separates: blouses or shirts tucked into a pair of wool-crepe pleat-fronted trousers or a pencil skirt look very smart but make sure tops are well-fitting and don't reveal too much cleavage. In cooler weather, a neat twinset or a fine-knit sweater are good alternatives and wearing a bright top beneath a navy or charcoal suit has an immediate visual impact. The shift dress has been a staple of the well-dressed woman's wardrobe for decades and still stands the test of time. If you don't wish to wear a suit, day in day out, many working women keep a versatile jacket on the back of their office chair for occasions when they need to quickly smarten up.

Should you work in a less conservative office, that still doesn't mean anything goes. Skinny jeans might be fine, but make them dark and team with a jacket, even if it is worn over a smart T-shirt rather than a shirt. Even in the most fashion-conscious offices, don't make the mistake of wearing see-through blouses or too-short skirts, although if your style generally errs towards the classic, you are unlikely to go wrong.

There are other questions as to what is acceptable that vary according to individual workplaces. Summer is the time when choices are most difficult to make – for example, are bare legs OK, or should you always wear tights (hosiery)? And while sandals with well-pedicured feet might be fine, flip-flops are a no-no as indeed are other more beach-friendly garments, such as spaghetti-strap tops. Be wary of displaying underwear, too – bra straps and visible panty lines are frankly off-putting in a meeting and when it comes to accessories and jewellery, less is definitely more.

The smartest shoes to wear are heels of some description. However, flats such as plain ballet-style pumps (so beloved of today's fashion designers that there are hundreds of versions to choose from) or even loafers or brogues with a nod to the recent trend in preppy, masculine-style touches can be equally smart. In winter, quality leather boots are a good alternative. Carrying a pair of heels in your bag is still commonplace, but please make the flats for walking a pair of smart-ish pumps rather than trainers (sneakers). It should go without saying but shoes for a smart working outfit must always be polished and in good condition. A good idea for the working woman is to keep polish and a cloth in your desk drawer to smarten up occasionally, and you might also keep hairspray and a little sewing kit or spare pair of tights.

The well-dressed woman should have little in her wardrobe that would not be acceptable in most workplaces but the key is always to judge each office by its own rules. If in doubt, err on the side of too smart rather than too casual. It is revealing that in some offices where almost anything goes, many women still choose to wear smarter clothes or suits, which can instil greater individual confidence and workplace credibility.

EVENINGWEAR

A HISTORY OF EVENINGWEAR

The twenty-first-century Cinderella is a lucky woman: her choice of eveningwear is far less restricted than that of her ancestors who, over the past 300 years since the advent of formal evening gowns in the nineteenth century, had to conform to a much stricter etiquette. In the Middle Ages there was not a specific dress to be worn for formal occasions (though an extra train might be added to everyday dresses) and what springs to mind when we imagine grand gowns of the past was inspired by the extravagant eighteenth-century court dress of the grandest royal houses of Europe. In the court of Versailles, where Marie Antoinette set costume trends that soon reverberated among other European courts, the instantly recognizable gown with its tightly fitting bodice, exaggerated wide skirt (panniers reached widths of an incredible 3.6 m/12 ft on occasion!) and train, all made of the finest Parisian fabrics, became the precedent for ostentatious style. Marie Antoinette was the original fashion model and first to bring court dress to the attention of the wider world through the work of early designers, such as Rose Bertin (1747–1813).

This courtly dress soon evolved into the popular sack-back gown with its box-pleated back, front opening to reveal a decorative "stomacher" or triangular panel of fabric, and wide-hoop skirt beneath the petticoat. A template for the evening gown was firmly established. Society's fashionable elite was quick to adopt the new gowns with subtle changes marking the most up-to-date designs. For example, during Queen Victoria's reign, formerly ankle-length gowns dropped to sweep the floor. In the 1830s, voluminous sleeves were in vogue; the 1840s saw a trend for off-the-shoulder, widely-flounced gowns, with necklines scooped ever-lower so that by the 1850s and 60s, they barely covered the bosom. Yet as the century drew to a close, the gown became longer and leaner, the décolletage squared and the wasp waist gained in popularity, often with the re-emergence of the over-sized train.

The twentieth century is when evening gowns became closer to how we envisage them today, though. From the 1920s, modernizers in the fashion world played with variations, from the Empire line, dropped waists and simple styles of the Flapper era to the tiny-waisted 1950s "New Look" gown famously created by Christian Dior to the understated gowns popularized by Jean Muir in the 1960s. Hem lengths waxed and waned, landing mid-calf or dropping to the ankle and since the advent of cocktail dresses, knee-length (or shorter) has become acceptable if not the norm, as opposed to a longer-length dress.

And finally, and perhaps most importantly for those who appreciate a little sartorial security, we have Coco Chanel to thank for popularizing black as a colour for eveningwear. Formal black was reserved for mourning and pale colours – even white – were the most popular, partly because only the very wealthy could afford a colour that spoiled so easily. Chanel's fondness for black and the extensive use of it in her designs was a precurser to that ubiquitous stalwart of every modern woman's wardrobe: the Little Black Dress (LBD).

Today, of course, it is almost unheard of to wear a floor-length evening gown to anything but the stiffest gatherings, to which most of us receive few invitations. And even on the most formal state occasion, it is clear that the various generations follow different rules – the Duchess of Cambridge, for example, does not routinely wear white gloves with her evening gowns. Despite the lack of formality there are still rules, albeit more flexible ones, to follow in order to always appear well dressed. With looser interpretations to dress codes, it is always essential to assess each occasion on its own merits, whatever is printed on the invitation. For example, instructions to wear a "lounge suit" to a wedding might make a knee-length printed, silk wraparound style dress, heels and jewels appropriate whereas the same code for a fortieth birthday party means a Little Black Dress is more likely to fit in.

WHITE TIE

This refers to full evening dress (named after the white bow tie that men would wear accompanied by a full tail coat) and is the most formal of dress codes. Usually, it is reserved for state occasions. This really does not allow much leeway from the full-length ball gown and best jewels; even a tiara is often required! The dress is traditionally considered correct only after 6 pm.

BLACK TIE

Where once accompanying a man in a dinner jacket would mean a woman should be similarly smartly dressed in a long gown this dress code has become more flexible over the years, so gauge each individual occasion and you will find that sometimes a shorter dress is acceptable. It should, however, be seen as an opportunity to wear a far smarter dress than to a simple cocktail party and it is advisable to choose a colour other than black. Similarly, dresses in traditional evening gown fabrics such as silk or satin or even chiffon or velvet, as the seasons dictate, are called for. Jewellery is essential and more attention should be paid to details such as matching shoes and bag than at a less formal occasion.

LOUNGE SUITS

Next in line down in formality from Black Tie, this has become a popular dress code for occasions such as weddings for it has become widely acknowledged that the modern man does not always have a dinner suit in his wardrobe. An ordinary suit for men equates to a smart dress for women but there is flexibility over length and personal style. Here, a cocktail dress or tea dress (see below) are perfectly acceptable options and while black is sometimes a controversial choice for some celebratory occasions such as weddings (and why not wear colour or print when you have the chance?), a Little Black Dress would not be out of place.

COCKTAIL

A cocktail dress is appropriate for semi-formal and some Back-Tie occasions. It is often assumed that

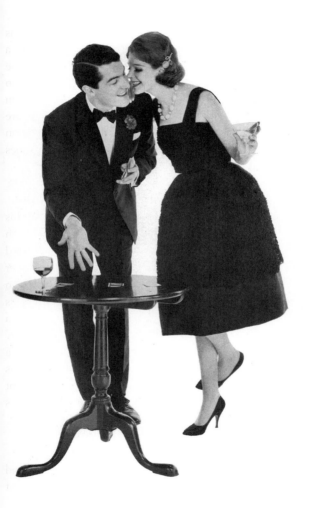

a cocktail dress is fitted and falls to just above the knee but this should be modified according to the style that best suits an individual. It is the perfect occasion to wear the little black dress. Cocktail does not necessarily refer to an evening event – cocktail dresses or fitted ladylike dress suits might equally be worn for a late afternoon smart event.

TEA DRESS

Originally designed as a woman's "at-home" dress for informal entertaining, the tea dress or gown was fashionable from the late nineteenth until the mid-twentieth century but this style has resurfaced in popularity and may be suitable for some evening occasions, particularly in summer. Essentially, it is a less structured dress and often in a light fabric with a pleasingly aesthetic print.

LITTLE BLACK DRESS

As arbiter of style and legendary fashion designer Christian Dior once wrote: "A little black frock is essential to every woman's wardrobe". And he was right – there are few such useful dresses that come in styles for all occasions. When it comes to choosing the perfect LBD for eveningwear, err on the side of smarter with a fabric such as silk or silk/satin, perhaps with spaghetti straps and almost always falling only to the knee or just below in the mould of the slash-necked shift so beloved of Audrey Hepburn. For such a wardrobe staple, it is essential to find a style with longevity that fits perfectly. To this end the Little Black Dress should be viewed as an investment piece, where it is worth paying for quality.

SMART/CASUAL

This is a rather ambiguous dress code, which can be loosely interpreted as neat and well-presented but not overly formal. For an evening occasion, a simple dress or a pair of smart trousers (not jeans) and a blouse or neat sweater, perhaps with heels, would suffice.

SHOES

A HISTORY OF SHOES

Shoes have been worn for many thousands of years, the earliest sandals dating as far back as 8,000 BC. The oldest leather shoe is believed to date to 3,500 BC and physical anthropologists have noted as long ago as 40,000 years that the middle toe bones of some human skeletons appear thinner, leading them to speculate that shoes were being worn even then (when walking barefoot, the middle toe is used for traction and is therefore relatively thick). Inevitably, few specimens have survived, the tanned skin of an animal not being a particularly long-lasting material.

It seems plausible then that shoes were first invented as a means of protecting the feet from the elements, although equally important reasons for early shoe-wearing included superstition, when wearing the skin of a killed animal was thought to harness its energy for future hunting success, and mythological beliefs – for example, in ancient Greece people believed that by wearing sandals, they were protected from Hades. Lastly, shoes were of course worn for decorative purposes. The

role of shoes as an indicator of status developed
very early on in the ancient worlds of Greece, Rome
and Egypt. Most footwear was not particularly
ostentatious – commoners wore plain wood, felt
or linen sandals – but the wealthy and influential
used decorative discs as well as gilt, embroidery
and pearls to customize their leather sandals,
which were also dyed a variety of natural colours,
including scarlet, saffron yellow, vermillion and
green. There were several fashions, some with
the bare minimum of simple straps at the toe and
ankle; others had ties reaching up to the calf.

Other shoes, some almost slipper-like and made
from luxurious fabrics such as silk and lavishly
embroidered or decorated with pearls, were popular
for indoor wear among the wealthy in ancient
Greece and a common practice was the ceremonial
lacing of matrimonial wedding shoes to symbolize
the new bride's commitment. Remarkably, in
ancient Rome and Egypt, there were even high-
heels – mostly in the shape of platform sandals or
ceremonial shoes.

The range of shoes commonly worn expanded to
include sandals, boots, clogs, slippers and of course
high platform heels by the Middle Ages. Again,
status determined which kind of shoe an individual

might wear. Members of the medieval Italian courts wore delicate silk or velvet shoes whereas peasants had clogs made of wood or cork. Heels became excessive in this era – for example, the *pianelle* and the Venetian *chopine*, a staggeringly high platform shoe, the highest recorded being a staggering 61 cm (24 in), which was popular in Europe between the fourteenth and seventeenth centuries. The thickness of sole was said to indicate a person's status and competition became so fierce that both Church and State were forced to intervene with legislation limiting the trend, further condemned by the well-documented association between the chopine and the courtesan.

By the eighteenth century, platforms fell from popularity – partly for the purely practical reason that the streets were becoming cleaner (previously, platforms had been worn to elevate their wearers from the filth flowing in the streets, among other reasons). The French led the way with a trend for smaller, more delicate shoes. Satin, silk and brocade were common, as were elaborate buckles of silver, gold and bronze, for men as well as women. By the nineteenth century, French fashion again set the styles, this time abandoning the heels and buckles of courtly shoes in favour of simple forms with a narrow, elongated shape, a black or white upper and pale leather within, often decorated with a rosette.

In the Victorian era, dainty, ankle-revealing slippers were replaced by the fashion for tightly laced up, often black, button-boots – an appropriate metaphor for the strict social mores of the time and naturally in keeping with the prolonged mourning of Queen Victoria for her husband Albert. Silk and velvet shoes were still worn for evening, though. In the Edwardian period, they once more became popular and styles were usually pointed: some high-cut with buttons up to the ankle; others lower, with a single buttoned strap. For evening, they had a rectangular, decorative buckle at the toe. Surprisingly, in the 1890s, heels rose with some reaching as high as 15 cm (6 in), though this had dropped by the turn of the twentieth century.

The twentieth century began with small-heeled delicate pumps for daywear but by the time the First World War broke out in 1914, comfort and practicality were the watchwords. Boots were back and even shoes became sturdier and wider across the toe. Following the end of the war, hemlines rose and with shoes now on display, footwear became more important. Buckles, feathers, rosettes, fur, ribbons and lace were all used to adorn newly revealed shoes. In the 1920s, along with Flapper dresses, pointed shoes became popular again and by the end of the decade, the heavy utilitarian styles of the war years were forgotten as fabrics lightened and colour became rife.

Shoe styles as we recognize them today really came into being in the 1930s. Women began to wear tailored suits, which required appropriate shoes; heels were lower and more angular and ankle straps became common. Two-tone, brogue-like styles were also popular, some laced in the "Oxford" style. Sandals also began to appear, particularly the fashionable "T-strap". Open-sided sandals and plain tennis pumps were required for outdoor leisure activities.

With the advent of the Second World War, footwear in the 1940s became difficult to procure and expensive to buy, forcing women to abandon fashion in favour of classic shoes that would last for years. Styles including the "Mary Jane", with its single strap across the foot and low heel, were popular, as were the lace-up Oxfords, which remained popular into the 1950s. By the end of the war, however, the mood was jubilant and fashion became similarly playful. The conservative shoes of wartime gave way to the high-heeled peep toe, sling-backed pumps that we so associate with late-1940s fashion.

Classic court shoes, ballet pumps and strappy sandals were mainstays of the chic 1950s female, but there was one arrival that has remained popular ever since: the stiletto heel. Versions of a pin-thin heel had been around since the late nineteenth century, but the stiletto's invention is usually attributed to the designer Roger Vivier who, in collaboration with Christian Dior to complement his celebrated "New Look" collection, created the perfect low-cut shoe. Barely covering the toe and instep, it was supported by a dagger-like, exaggeratedly slender heel. First mentioned in the press in 1953, the style was revolutionary and became an instant success, perfectly in keeping with the ladylike fashions of the 1950s.

Both chunky and heeled knee-high boots became extremely fashionable during the 1960s and '70s, while super-high stiletto heels further enhanced the impact of the micro-miniskirt. The feminist movement was less keen on the stiletto, claiming it objectified women and furthermore (literally, as well as metaphorically), crippled them. Alternative shoes with squat square heels became popular until the arrival of the platform in the 1970s, with some designs rivalling the Venetian chopine in their extraordinary height.

Taking us up to the present day, the 1980s and 1990s saw a revival in high heels, although this time for the emancipated woman. A pair of spike heels was the ultimate power shoe, symbolizing "yuppie" success as well as excess. As the century drew to a close, Manolo Blahnik and Jimmy Choo became household names and gradually, shoe choices widened. Ballet pumps and flat driving shoes answer the call for style and comfort, stilettos remain popular while chunkier heels and moulded platform soles also feature regularly in designers' collections. Trainers (sneakers) hit their stride in these years, becoming generally more acceptable; they were also designer items (and often expensive) in their own right.

SHOE TYPES

These days there is no one fashion. However for the well-dressed lady certain types of shoe afford more elegance than others. Listed following are different styles for different occasions.

BALLET PUMP

Nowadays, ballet flats are unbelievably popular. Beloved of stars such as Audrey Hepburn and Brigitte Bardot, they are ubiquitous when paired with skinny jeans among off-duty models and actresses, but are just as suitable for the traditionally elegant older woman. From the classic Chanel quilted pump with its contrast colour toe and little bow to a thoroughly modern brightly coloured patent pair, it is possible to have an entire wardrobe of ballet pumps. They are one of the most versatile, not to mention comfortable shoes to include in the well-dressed lady's wardrobe.

DRIVING SHOE

Extremely popular in the 1990s and early 2000s, the driving shoe popularized by the Italian leather brand Tod's has been somewhat usurped by the ballet pump as the off-duty shoe of choice. That said, the driving shoe with its overall higher structure and a more squared-off toe is a better fit

for some women. Trademark little studs at the heel
and on the soft sole make for a Euro-chic look that
is just as versatile as the ballet flat.

COURT SHOE OR PUMP

This is a catchall term for slip-in, low-fronted
smart shoes with a heel. The variety of pumps on
the market is extraordinary, with designs in colours
and prints, peep toes or sling-backs, kitten heels
or super-high stilettos; some have a rounded toe,
others are sharply pointed. A pair of black high-
heeled pumps, perhaps in patent leather, is a
useful addition to the well-dressed lady's wardrobe
and excellent paired with tailored suits or pencil
skirts for the office.

LOAFER

The loafer has seen a rise in popularity of late,
previously being associated somewhat with the
preppy look of the 1980s and early 1990s. But for
women who find ballet flats too insubstantial or
prefer a slightly more androgynous look, this slip-
in shoe – traditionally with a band across the front
into which was slipped a penny coin, hence the
original term "penny loafer" – is a fine alternative.
A black, brown or tan leather pair looks equally
good with slim trousers, dark jeans or even tailored
shorts in summer.

BROGUE
The brogue is another traditionally masculine shoe that has been adopted by women. Flat, with laces and usually stitching detail on the uppers, a pair of simple brogues has an elegant androgyny about it and can be worked into several different looks. For example, caramel brogues paired with dark denim jeans and a tailored jacket, or black brogues with slim tailored black trousers and a blouse and, in summer, pale cream brushed leather or suede brogues suit a vintage-feel floral dress.

OXFORDS
Fashionable from the 1930s to the 1950s, the Oxford is basically similar to the brogue although it may have high heels. Laces are the essential detail.

MARY JANES
These pumps have a rounded toe and a characteristic strap across the ankle. Usually low-heeled, they may be high on occasion – a chunky, platform-heeled version has recently become popular. On balance, the Mary Jane is not so elegant as a plain pump, though.

PLATFORM HEEL
As the name suggests, this is a heel that raises the whole sole of a shoe. Famously associated with the

1970s, lately a modified version has once again become fashionable, with a more elegantly moulded sole and inverted-triangle heel. High-heeled pumps in this new style certainly have a place in the well-dressed lady's wardrobe, particularly as an easier-to-walk-in alternative to the stiletto.

STILETTO HEEL
Popular since the early 1950s, the stiletto is a super-thin high heel on a pump or sandal. Eternally fashionable, though it can look somewhat trashy if paired with inelegant clothes, the stiletto is a mainstay of evening outfits in particular.

KITTEN HEEL
This is a short, slim heel, very like a stiletto but with a slightly bulbous base; popular in the 1950s on pointed court shoes. This is a very elegant and versatile shoe, beloved of Audrey Hepburn.

SLING-BACK
As suggested by the name, sling-backs have a strap that runs around the back of the ankle rather than a fully moulded piece. The style has been popular since the 1930s and appears on many different types of shoe, including pumps and sandals. A kitten- or high-heeled satin or leather sling-back pump is a useful alternative to the full court version.

BOOTS

Unless you are fortunate enough to live in a highly temperate climate, boots are an essential part of most women's wardrobes. Originally popularized by Queen Victoria and the norm beneath the voluminous crinoline skirts of the nineteenth century, different versions have been popular ever since. Fashion has run the gamut through the knee-high stilettos of the 1960s, 1970s clumpy platform soles, glittery boots for frenzied disco-goers, "Moon" boots, "Biker" boots and Doc Martens in the 1980s. And let's not forget the overwhelming success of the comfortable sheepskin run-arounds from Australia and New Zealand, the Ugg boot and its competitors – finally given fashion credibility in a collaboration with Jimmy Choo in 2011.

If you plan to invest in just a few pairs, however, the most useful styles for the well-dressed lady are either a classic knee-high leather pair in a riding style (tan, brown or black, either flat or with a slight heel – this is good for skirts or over skinny jeans for a more casual look) and a shorter, black ankle boot with a kitten or narrow heel that may be worn for smarter occasions with formal black trousers.

SANDALS

These days it would be possible to fill a couple of shoe racks full of sandals: cork wedges, brightly coloured flip-flops, bejewelled high heels, strappy snakeskin sling-backs with moulded platforms, Grecian-style rope flats, the list goes on. But summer is the one time when you can remain elegant while embracing more exotic colours, prints and fabrics. As long as you keep your clothes in the classic mould, there is no reason not to indulge yourself.

TRAINERS (SNEAKERS)

Though fashionable, designer-labelled and even cult-inspiring (not to mention expensive), sports shoes are never an elegant choice for day-to-day wear and really do belong in the gym. Otherwise, the only trainer that belongs in the wardrobe of the well-dressed lady is the simple white plimsoll (Keds), maybe with some subtle blue piping, and it is strictly for off-duty days. Peeping out from under a pair of wide-leg linen trousers and topped with a striped Breton top, they have a certain Chanel-like style.

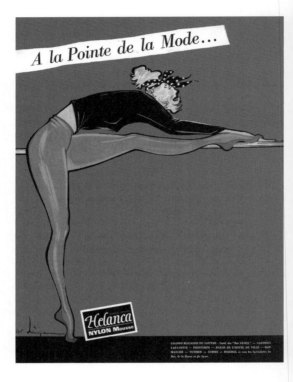

A 1960s advertisement for "skintight" Gehel pantyhose.

SOCKS AND HOSIERY

A HISTORY OF SOCKS AND HOSIERY

Like shoes, socks have been worn to keep the feet warm and protected for several thousand years. In fact, the word "sock" is derived from the Latin word *soccus* – the term for a loose-fitting slipper worn by comic actors in ancient Rome, which then became the Olde English *socc* and the Middle English word *socke*. The first makeshift socks, which archaeologists believe date back as far as the Stone Age, were made of animal skins, gathered and tied at the ankles; the ancient Greeks also used the warmth of matted animal hair to create basic socks and the Romans wore leather and woven fabric socks. Later, socks became popular among Europe's religious, where they were seen to protect purity and by 1,000 AD, they began to symbolize wealth among the nobility.

During the Middle Ages a version of tights (hose), as we now recognize them, first appeared, initially referring simply to garments for men. The term "hose" was a general one, meaning any style of clothing that covered the legs and lower body, but by the seventeenth century, the term had been replaced by breeches (garments running from the waist down to the knee or just below and worn over stockings). Until the sixteenth century, stockings covered the foot and leg but were open at the crotch. A cod-piece was also worn, both to cover ill-disguised genitalia and allow men to relieve themselves. Henry VIII popularized large padded cod-pieces but the trend had died out by the seventeenth century.

In the early days, stockings were made of woven cloth. However, the invention of the knitting machine (originally known as the "stocking frame") by William Lee in 1589 meant that woollen stockings could be quickly made as they were by now a clothing staple for both sexes. Denied a patent for his invention by Queen Elizabeth (who considered woollen stockings to be unattractive), Lee developed his machine to enable him to make fine silk stockings. There is no conclusive evidence that he ever received a patent for this particular invention either, but once the Industrial Revolution took hold in the early 1800s, cloth-making machines were needed for the new factories. In 1864, William Cotton introduced a new and improved version of Lee's original design. Finally, circular knitting machines able to produce knitted cloth in a tube shape – perfect for stockings and tights – had been developed.

Until the 1920s, hosiery was worn purely for warmth; dresses were long and legs rarely revealed. But with the Flapper fashions of the 1920s and rising hemlines, women began wearing stockings to cover their exposed legs. Initially, they were made of silk but in the early part of the twentieth century, the manmade fabric rayon (or "viscose", as it later became known) was invented. This artificial silk was popular during the 1930s until it was superseded by nylon in 1940.

Nylon was hugely successful as it did not bag and sag, unlike silk and rayon stockings (which frequently did), and added a shiny allure to women's legs. By 1942 the demand for nylon for war purposes (for example, parachute making) was so great that stockings were virtually unobtainable for most women and, as a consequence, the black market thrived. Women unable to get hold of stockings would paint a fake seam line down the back of their legs to give the impression that they were wearing a pair, all the while hoping not to get caught in the rain and have the line run!

Until the end of the 1950s, women always wore stockings (which ended at the thigh and were held up by a suspender belt), but in the early 1960s Lycra began to be added. This improved the fit and most liberating of all, allowed for the invention of the first tights – or "pantyhose". Literally a pair of panties and stockings sewn together ("panty" and "hose"), they were an immediate hit. The production technique was quickly perfected, allowing the new pantyhose to become seamless just in time for the fashion for the miniskirt. This was also the decade in which Mary Quant is credited with inventing playful coloured and patterned tights, making them a fashion item, too. The terms "pantyhose" and "tights" are not quite interchangeable – in the US, "pantyhose" refers to lighter denier, usually nude seamless tights, whereas "tights" means darker, opaque or woollen versions. In the UK, the term "tights" is universally used.

SOCKS AND HOSIERY – WHAT TO WEAR

Tights, stockings and variations such as hold-ups (self-supporting stockings) are a staple part of women's wardrobes today and have become a fashionable accessory in their own right. Once plain and discreet, socks are often deliberately colourful, printed or worn poking out of the top of boots.

AMERICAN TAN PANTYHOSE

When it comes to tights, there are strong opinions particularly when it comes to whether it is acceptable to wear American tan or should one stick to sheer black. As with most things, fashion plays a part. For many years, tan tights were seen as the preserve of the stuffy and matronly until inimitably stylish women such as France's former First Lady Carla Bruni and Kate Middleton, Duchess of Cambridge, began wearing them and a new trend was sparked. Of course these women operate under different protocols to the rest of us. Nevertheless, nude or tan tights have experienced a revival from the no-man's land of fashion.

When it comes to tights, judge each outfit on its merits. If you can get away with bare legs for a summer occasion, this is better than tan tights but if the occasion is very smart or you are going to work, nude tights with a colourful, pale or lightweight dress are more appropriate than black. Pale matt are usually a better choice than shiny or deeply tan "wooden legs" versions, which are a bit too 1980s in feel.

BLACK SHEER TIGHTS

A stalwart addition to the well-dressed woman's wardrobe, you should own several pairs in different deniers. Excellent with dresses and suits and even sheer pop-socks are acceptable beneath tailored trousers. Always carry a spare pair in case of ladders and holes. Navy is appropriate if you are a wearing navy tailored suit, for example.

OPAQUE WOOLLEN TIGHTS

Another controversy is whether opaque thick woollen tights are something of a godsend or hark back rather too much to school uniform days. Certainly they are warm and highly flattering to the leg; if you choose carefully, they can look good in winter with a skirt and boots. Super-fine wool or failing that, 100-denier matt nylon tights, are the most elegant choices.

PRINTED TIGHTS

The trend for printed sheer tights shows no sign of abating and while they can add interest and a certain chic *joie de vivre* to an outfit, careful selection is essential. Subtle prints on sheer black tights are fine but a garish leopard-printed pair should be avoided at all costs. Brands such as Wolford, with a history of high-quality production, are best and last longer, rather than cheaper copies that have jumped on the fashion bandwagon. Keep the rest of your outfit simple: for example, a classic black dress with statement sheer black patterned tights.

TIGHTS AND SANDALS

This is a tricky call. Unless you really can't (or won't) go out with bare legs (for example, when attending a very formal occasion, although closed shoes would be more appropriate here anyway), tights and sandals are a no-no. They are fine with a pair of sling-backs (preferably with a closed toe), although beware of the ankle-strap slipping off the nylon. A tiny peep toe might be fine but tights worn with strappy stilettos simply looks bad.

SOCKS

Once plain, black, blue or beige, socks made from cotton or some manmade fibre were never to be revealed. Now jeans are rolled up to display brightly coloured or striped socks, over-the-knee versions are paired with short skirts and socks designed specially for Wellington boots are big business. These are mostly fashion trends for the well-dressed lady in search of classic style to avoid. By all means treat yourself to soft, well-fitting socks to wear with your loafers or brogues, even striped ones as a personal style quirk but not actually on display. As for the trend shown on some designer catwalks for socks and sandals paired with skirts, unless you happen to be a teenage model, forget it or you will look like a mad old bag lady!

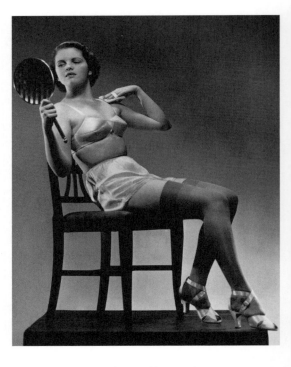

Matching cami-knickers and bra for the 1950s woman.

LINGERIE

A HISTORY OF UNDERWEAR

Today we take the modesty and hygiene that underwear affords us for granted, albeit with acceptance of its erotic connotations, so it is difficult to comprehend that women did not even wear underwear, or certainly not knickers (panties), until the nineteenth century.

In ancient Rome a type of loincloth or shorts known as a *subligaculum* was worn by both sexes and women sometimes wore a band of cloth (*stophium*) around their upper body. During the Middle Ages men might sometimes wear a pair of linen shorts but the only undergarment worn by women was a long linen undershirt, known as a "shift". By the sixteenth century, the Elizabethan fashion for extremely rigid bodices meant that corsets, a version of which had already become popular, began to be stiffened by the use of whalebone and the tightly laced corset soon became an indispensable garment as it gave bodices a much-admired, geometrically straight line.

Over the next few centuries, however, the use of an increased strength of corsetry, certain styles even involving steel or iron as well as whalebone, led to a fashion for a unnatural female form and much suffering. The waist was cinched into an impossibly small circumference, the hips forced into a similarly unnatural shape and the bust pushed high, towards the chin. As one commentator wrote in the early nineteenth century, their form moulded one into "the body of an ant"! Women could barely breathe, they were unable to bend and soon their back muscles became so deformed that they required "stays" to stand upright. In our modern age of comfortable clothes, it is hard to imagine the crippling pain that these women experienced. Digestion was difficult, stomach pains the norm and most distressing of all, there were specially designed pregnancy corsets, which often resulted in miscarriages or birth defects.

Nevertheless, the hourglass figure (and the corset required to maintain it) remained popular throughout the Victorian era (worn beneath fashionable crinoline frames) into the Edwardian era, when bustles and bum-pads were used to create an exaggeratedly prominent rear. The design of the corset was short or long, according to fashion, and hose supporters began to appear at the base, to which stockings were attached. By then, women were wearing voluminous "drawers" – drawstring cotton, silk or linen undergarments that reached their knees. For practical purposes, these precursors to knickers were not closed at the crotch for it would have been nigh on impossible to climb out of so many layers of clothing to relieve oneself!

As with so many women's fashions, it was the two world wars that finally ended the reign of the corset. The beginning of the twentieth century also saw voluminous drawers, with delicate buttoned openings for a woman to relieve herself without undressing, replaced by closed knickers or panties. During the First World War, women expected to replace men at work simply could not wear corsets while performing manual tasks and the Flapper era that followed saw a marked change, with loose dresses all the rage. Although the 1930s saw a revival of the "wasp-waist" look, the Second World War again made restrictive clothing impractical. The "New Look" of the 1950s did accentuate the waist once more but by now the whalebone corset had been usurped by a variety of girdles made from elastic fabric. Reaching to the waist, the "panty-girdle" had straps to attach suspenders; other types of girdle extended over the breasts and were known as "corselletes".

Throughout the 1960s, the panty-girdle remained popular but with the invention of tights, it became less necessary and gradually the trend for accentu- ating the waist waned. While today a variety of control pants are still worn on occasion, the daily forcing of one's body into an uncomfortable, artificial shape is unappealing to most women.

Versions of the brassière (or bra) first appeared in the late nineteenth century and the original patent for a bra in the US was granted to Mary Phelps Jacob in 1914. It was not until the 1930s that bras began to be produced on a larger scale and at this time the letters of the alphabet were used to describe different cup sizes. Bra fashions changed in tandem with clothes fashions – for example, in the 1950s companies such as Berlei, Triumph and Marks & Spencer created circular, stitched bras that gave women the all-important conical look beneath their close-fitting sweaters, a trend sparked by Howard Hughes' obsession with Jane Russell's breasts, for which he designed a prototype underwire bra for maximum uplift. In the 1960s, women's libbers may have demanded you "burn your bra", but for many women the support became indispensable, with the average bra size increasing rapidly (in the 1950s, the average woman wore a B-cup, today one brand catering to larger sizes – Bravissimo – has gone up as far as an L-cup!). It is now estimated between 75 and 95 per cent of the world's women wear bras regularly.

Over the last few decades, bras have become fashion items as much as practical garments and the variety is ever-increasing; 1964 saw the invention of the Wonderbra and since then, these garments have evolved to include seamless fabrics for beneath T-shirts, moulded-cups, padded-cups, push-up bras and bras for plunge necklines, halter-necks and strapless outfits. Even modern versions of the girdle and corset are enjoying a revival – sometimes worn as outerwear as much as underwear – confirming that in the twentieth century, lingerie is big business.

FINDING THE RIGHT BRA

It is estimated that 80 per cent of women are wearing the wrong bra size. The best way to determine your size is to be professionally measured, however there is a formula you can use at home: first, measure beneath your bust around your back (reasonably tightly but not uncomfortably so). This is your back size (if measuring in inches, round up to an even number). Some home guides advise adding 13 cm (5 in) to this measurement to gauge your bra size, but this is ludicrous and would never give adequate support. Bear in mind that most women wear far too large a back size.

Next, measure across the bust and the difference indicates your cup size – for example, if you are 5 cm (2 in) larger across the bust, you will measure an A cup; 7.5 cm (3 in) larger is a B cup; 10 cm (4 in) is a C cup; and 12 cm (5 in) difference equals a D cup. Remember, if you go up a back size, the cup size is proportionally bigger, too – so, if you feel the 32D is too tight, a 34C might be better. Of course, your bra size can change if you lose or gain weight, or become pregnant. Bear in mind that bras are supposed to feel tight, not red-welt-inducing but tighter than a lot of women are used to wearing them. In order to see if the bra fits properly, practise the "swoop and scoop" method: put the shoulder straps of the new bra on, then lean forward and scoop up the breasts before fastening the back (the tightest fastening to begin with as, over time, bras tend to stretch).

Now stand up and scoop your breasts from beneath to ensure they are properly encased in the cups. There should be no bulging at the side of the cups and minimal bulging beneath the back although if you have a fleshy back, some bulge is inevitable and this does not mean the bra is necessarily too small. The top of the cup should lie flat against the bust with no gape – if you are fuller at the bottom of your breasts (a natural consequence of ageing, childbearing and breastfeeding), choose a bra that is cut lower – for example, a plunge or balcony bra. A moulded cup is a good idea for almost all women to improve their shape and bras are so cleverly designed these days that even padded ones are discreet and can help give a better shape, even if you don't need the extra size.

YOUR CAPSULE COLLECTION

For everyday wear, nothing beats a simple, nude, flat-seamed, moulded-cup bra that is invisible below even the finest white T-shirt. A black version is another good choice for beneath fine knitwear. White "T-shirt" bras, as they are known, actually show up underneath white T-shirts (which is why a nude colour is a better choice), but white bras are pretty, particularly with lace, and work well under blouses and shirts. Other than that, the world is your oyster. Many women enjoy wearing beautiful underwear under the plainest business suit and there are plenty of exquisite versions around in different colours, with various trims, embroidery, lace and ribbons. No truly chic woman would ever say that underwear doesn't count!

When it comes to knickers (panties), personal preference again plays a part. Many young women prefer G-strings to avoid the unattractive panty-line but if your trousers are not super-tight, there is no reason not to wear well-cut briefs, in black, white or nude.

Buy new knickers and bras often, ideally every six months, as baggy, greying ones should not be part of the well-dressed woman's wardrobe and in an appropriate size – bulges around the bottom are simply not attractive. Bear in mind that control pants are amazing these days and even if not worn daily, are useful on occasion. There are a variety of brands available but the market-leader is Spanx, with its vast array of styles and celebrity endorsements. Lastly, as with bras, there are endless knickers for those who appreciate pretty underwear, although many of these are expensive. Whenever possible, buy and wear matching sets of bras and knickers, to ensure a well-dressed look from skin-layer outwards.

The Bra that launched the American look

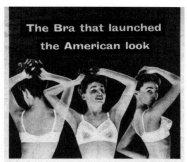

The Playtex Living Bra fits and feels as if fashioned for you alone.

Every day, everywhere, women are saying

"Never before such heavenly comfort"

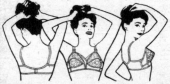

Study these pictures. Detail by wonderful detail. Special elastic back sets lower, stays lower. Never rides up. Superbly comfortable. Moves and breathes with you, never against you. Always. However active you may be.

Consider the elastic criss-cross front. Notice how low it dips. Dividing oh, so divinely! Supporting you oh, so superbly! And see how the sculptured nylon gently cups and ups. Moulding your figure *the way you want.*

Another exclusive Playtex feature — the bias-cut elastic sides. They never gape. Never cut. Self-adjust to your every movement. Hugging, holding you. Yet allowing blissful freedom. And such fabulous fit!

Tailored, gleaming white, elastic and nylon. Easy to wash, needs no ironing, never loses its perfect shape. 32 to 40. Cups: A, B and C. To fit every size and every in-between size.

27/6

Playtex LIVING BRA

© 1956 *TRADE MARK*

MADE AT PLAYTEX PARK, PORT GLASGOW, SCOTLAND. LONDON OFFICE: 17 STRATTON STREET, LONDON, W.I

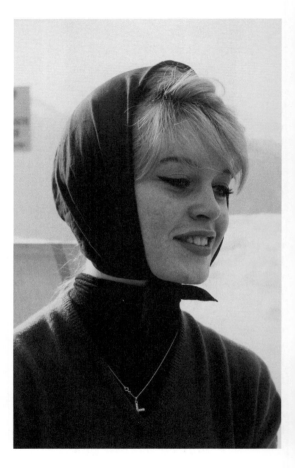

The chic headscarf on Brigitte Bardot, 1958.

SCARVES

A HISTORY OF SCARVES

One of the earliest examples of scarf-wearing is that of the finely woven scarf worn by the Egyptian Queen Nefertiti beneath her conical headdress; similarly ancient are the Chinese sculptures from 1,000 BC, which include rectangular, delicate, fringed pieces of cloth. Undoubtedly, scarves of different fabrics have been worn for thousands of years, by both sexes and for many different purposes. For example, in ancient Rome, a scarf known as a *sudarium* (translatable as "sweat cloth") was used by men to wipe the sweat from their necks and faces in hot weather; Egyptians used long scarf-like belts for an early form of belly-dancing and by the Middle Ages, gossamer scarves were first worn attached to the tip of a tall pointed hat in one of the first instances of scarves being a fashionable part of an outfit.

Also, in the Middle Ages it is thought scarves began to be used to differentiate the ranks of soldiers, first among Chinese warriors. Around the seventeenth century, Croatian mercenaries wore scarves to signify rank – officers wore silk whereas lower ranks were issued with cotton scarves. As a result of the Croatian habit of scarf wearing, the French adopted the term "cravat" (from the Croatian *kravata*) for men's scarves and it became popular to show allegiance to political parties by the colour of one's scarf.

Scarves have long been associated with customs, including an eighteenth-century New England habit, where the family of a deceased person gave away scarves to friends and other members of the community at the funeral ceremony. Over time, the custom became frowned upon as inappropriately extravagant during a time of mourning and in Massachusetts legislation was passed banning the practice at the end of the eighteenth century. Scarves remained popular gifts, however and legend has it that Napoleon Bonaparte sent his first wife Joséphine many luxurious cashmere versions from his travels in India.

It was during the early nineteenth century that scarves became a real fashion accessory for both men and women. Beethoven popularized the wearing of silk neck scarves beneath a dandyish suit and shirt. A few decades later, in 1837, the French company The Hermès Group was founded, although it would not be for another 100 years that Hermès moved from its origins as maker of harnesses, bridles and saddlery to retailing its iconic printed silk scarves.

In the same year, Queen Victoria came to the throne and further popularized the scarf, both as a fashionable accessory and as a means of differentiating between the social classes. Victorian scarves were elaborate and often made from embroidered or delicately knitted fabrics trimmed with lace and adorned with pearls. Shawls were large and provided both warmth and the finishing touches to an outfit; much smaller scarves, sometimes ruffled or arranged into a type of collar, were aslo worn. During the Edwardian era scarves remained popular, including the fashion for tying a scarf over the top of a large over-sized hat and then tying it beneath the chin to secure the headpiece.

The late Victorian, early Edwardian period also saw the emergence of the flamboyant feather boa and in the early twentieth century, the legendary dancer Isadora Duncan started a trend for similarly extravagant, long, silk-chiffon flowing scarves. Alas, this passion for long scarves ended her life in a freak accident when a scarf became entangled in the wheels of the car she was travelling in, instantly breaking her neck, in 1927.

Knitted scarves have always been popular and during the First World War, women were urged to "knit for victory", providing soldiers with homespun comfort from the cold. Similarly warm were the fur stoles and tippets popular in the 1930s. Printed silk scarves, the most iconic being those made by Hermès (which began production in 1937 and are still hugely popular today), have been worn by a roll-call of illustrious women, including Grace Kelly (who once used one as a stylish sling for her broken arm), Jackie Kennedy, HRH Queen Elizabeth II and more recently, Sarah Jessica Parker, Madonna and Sharon Stone (who notoriously used one for a bondage scene in the *Basic Instinct* movie!).

Today there are many different kinds of scarf for diverse purposes – for example, plaid woollen scarves of the type made famous by the British company Burberry were once only worn by gentlemen but are now just as common on women. Silk scarves are still hugely popular and endlessly versatile, while the late-1990s fashion for the oversized pashmina shawl shows no signs of abating.

Scarves   151

Types of Scarf

Adding a scarf is one of the easiest ways to update an outfit. Aside from the stalwart wool or cashmere winter scarf in a plain colour or plaid, there are endless lightweight knitted, crocheted, silk or modal scarves in fashionable prints and colours that can quickly smarten or modernize a basic shirt, T-shirt or dress. A statement scarf, casually wrapped around the neck, is an easy way to look on trend without having to spend a fortune on the latest designer fashion – although the best scarves are expensive.

Pashminas, originally used in Nepal for travel, warmth and basic survival, have become rather too ubiquitous and there are many poor imitations around that have no place in the well-dressed lady's wardrobe. However, an oversized, butter-soft cashmere scarf is an invaluable addition to your wardrobe. Worn, as it was intended, for warmth by folding in half to form a large triangle wrapped over the shoulders or folded and knotted about the neck, a fine-knit pashmina should never be bulky, just elegant.

Slippery square silk scarves, printed with a distinctive motif (often equestrian or military in feel, or with prestigious banners or coats of arms and usually with a border) can look somewhat dated, which is perhaps why there is such a current vogue for long, rectangular printed scarves in fabrics including rayon and chiffon. But these are, it must be remembered, iconic designs that have stood the test of time. Today, Hermès sells more scarves than ever before. Indeed, one estimate suggests in the holiday season in Paris, each Hermès store sells a scarf every 20 seconds! If your budget won't stretch to Hermès, plenty of other fashion houses, such as Liberty's of London or high street chains such as Marks & Spencer sell similarly good silk scarves and there are ways of tying a silk scarf that are utterly classic and extremely dignified (as well as helpful in disguising an ageing neck). There are younger, more fashionable ways to use this kind of scarf, although trends for wearing it as a halter-neck top, super-skimpy sarong or bandana might cause Pierre Hermès to turn in his grave!

BASIC WAYS TO TIE A SCARF

There are entire books devoted to tying scarves. However, for most women, a few options are enough.

BASIC LOOP AND PULL

This is by far the easiest method to use on rectangular scarves, either made from a long length of chiffon or silk, or a woollen scarf. Hold the scarf in the middle to create a double layer (you may need to fold a particularly wide scarf once or twice lengthways first) and hold behind your neck, then pull the two ends through the loop created by folding the scarf in two. Pull down for a simple, chic look. This also works for a pashmina if you fold it in half into a triangle first, then continue folding until you have a long, narrow rectangle.

UNSTRUCTURED WRAP

This method looks especially effective when using a printed lightweight scarf. With the vogue for less structured dressing, this slightly bohemian way of tying a scarf can nevertheless dress up an outfit nicely. Fold the scarf in half lengthwise if it is overly wide, or even just bunch it up slightly, then simply take the ends in each hand and place in front of your neck. Cross the two ends over behind your neck, then bring them back to the front, making sure the scarf is not too tight. Arrange the central loop and two ends so they look in proportion and fluff up the fabric to ensure it fills the neck.

SIMPLE SILK SQUARE NECK-SCARF
It is the printed silk scarf that can be tied in so many different ways, however the most traditional and neatest method is to fold two corners into the middle to make overlapping triangles. Now continue folding until you have a long rectangle, almost as narrow as a gentleman's tie. Next, place in front of your neck, cross over behind and bring the ends forward. Now tie a knot in the ends and arrange attractively (perhaps slightly off-centre) and leave as is or tuck the ends into the neck of a shirt, sweater or jacket. An alternative tie is to fold into a rectangle as before, then twist the scarf into a long rope and, beginning in front of the neck, take it behind, then cross once again in front and tie at the back. This will sit close to the neck, almost like a silk choker, and looks elegant as well as being very secure.

HEADSCARF
Famously beloved of 1950s icons such as Marilyn Monroe, the silk printed scarf worn over the head

is a retro look that is also practical. You may not have a lifestyle that calls for riding in open-top cars round the French Riviera or stalking wild birds on windy marshes but knowing how to tie a headscarf is still useful, if only for "bad hair" days. Choose a large enough square scarf, at least 75 x 75 cm (30 x 30 in), fold it into a triangle and place the long edge on top of your head, just slightly back from the start of the hairline. Now bring the edges beneath your chin and tie. The trick to avoiding the "Queen Mother" look and keeping it more Marilyn is to tie the knot well to the side, not centrally beneath the chin. This is also a lovely way to show off any pattern on your scarf. Pair with vintage oversized sunglasses for the ultimate in 1950s glamour.

THE COWBOY

A modish way to wear a neck wrap, this style is adaptable to many outfits and necklines.

1   Fold a square scarf into a triangle.
2   Turn over the folded edge.
3   Place the scarf in front of you with the point hanging straight down, then take the ends behind your neck, cross over, and bring to the front.
4   Tie the ends together at the front of the neck.

THE GRACE KELLY

This style is named for the famous Grace Kelly, who used this method of wearing a scarf to protect her hairstyle and still look magnificent. The instructions below are for a square scarf, but an oblong scarf can also be used.

1 Fold a square scarf into a triangle.
2 Place the scarf over the head with the folded edge facing forward.
3 Bring the folded corners down under the chin and cross them, pushing the points back around the neck on each side.
4 Tie the folded corners together at the nape of the neck, catching the loose corners of the scarf under the knot. Leave the ends loose.

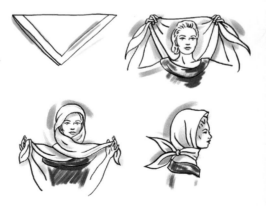

THE FRENCH TWIST

This elegant knot can be worn with almost any top and is ideal for filling in the neck of a suit, jacket or coat. If worn with a collared shirt, place the bow towards the middle instead of to the side.

1 Fold a square scarf into a bias band fold.
2 Centre the scarf behind your neck. Wrap around, crossing the ends in front of the neck and pull forward.
3 Tie a single knot centred underneath the chin then twist the scarf jauntily to one side of the neck so that the knot is off-centre.
4 Finish by tying a bow. Let the ends hang loosely.

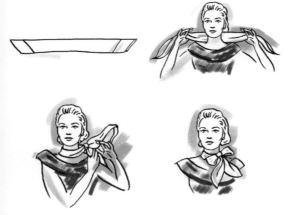

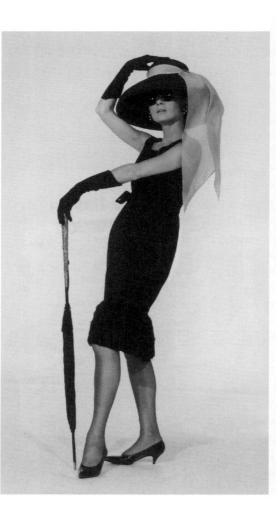

HATS

THE HISTORY OF HATS

It is a rare occasion these days that calls for a hat and at even the smartest of weddings being hat-less is not a cause for entrance to be barred. Consider the choice of British Prime Minister's wife Samantha Cameron to wear a discreet beaded piece rather than a hat when she attended the wedding ceremony of HRH Prince William and Kate Middleton at Westminster Abbey. For some, this was a terrible faux pas in etiquette terms while others, admiring her overall elegant outfit, had no complaints. In light of this it seems extraordinary that until the 1960s, hats formed an essential part of a well-dressed lady's outfit and in the first few decades of the twentieth century everyone, rich or poor, wore a hat (and usually gloves, too) simply to leave the house.

We have been covering our heads for thousands of years but the earliest practice was simply to pull animal skins over the head for protection; later, in ancient Greece and Rome, simple skullcaps appeared, including the "liberty cap" given to freed slaves. Women were expected to cover their heads but did so with veils, scarves, hoods, caps and wimples rather than structured hats, which did not appear until the end of the sixteenth century. The word "milliner" is first recorded in the sixteenth century and referred to retailers of haberdashery products from Milan (hence *Millaners*), which included gloves, ribbons, straw and other essentials for hat-making.

In the late seventeenth century women's hats became a distinct industry apart from men's headwear (the term "milliner" applies to those making hats for women; "hat-maker" for men). By the eighteenth century, Swiss and Italian straws, along with imitations made from materials as varied as horsehair, grass and cardboard, were moulded into hats and trimmed with velvet and tulle, as well as flamboyant feathers made by the *plumassiers*, whose business was the dyeing and arranging of feathers to adorn fashion items and also for use in interior decoration.

Hats became increasingly fashionable, with the bonnet dominating the early part of the nineteenth century (the larger, the better), trimmed with as many ribbons, flowers, feathers and any other attractive materials as the head could bear the weight of. During the Victorian era, hat and bonnet shapes changed from one year to the next and included the romantic wide-brimmed leghorn straw trimmed with lace, tulle or flowers (this style of hat was popularly worn by children) and slightly later, the emergence of the pillbox. Trimmings ranged from the ostentatious to the frankly bizarre, including small birds, beetles, fruits and vegetables. At the very end of the century, bonnets fell out of favour to be replaced by the wider-brimmed, ribbon-trimmed hats so redolent of the Edwardian era. These enormous creations, which required a good deal of engineering on the part of the milliner, remained popular until the First World War.

Wartime saw a relaxation of the Edwardian strictures that made even stepping out of the house without a hat and gloves a serious breach of etiquette, but hat wearing remained the norm. In the 1920s, fashion switched to straight, unstructured long dresses and chemise-like tops, perfectly suited to the new fashionable headwear: the cloche hat. This elegant design, moulded to the head and an ideal companion to the radical new, boyish bobbed hairstyle was beloved of stars such as the showgirl Louise Brooks. But the 1930s saw a backlash against the head-hugging cloche and wider-brimmed curved hats came back into vogue, often worn tilted dramatically to one side of the head. For truly bad-hair days an elegant turban – à la designer Elsa Schiaparelli – sufficed as stylish headgear.

Hats remained an essential part of an outfit during the Second World War and the 1940s, although rationing affected size. They were often smaller, with a single feather trim; utilitarian berets and scarves knotted into a headband were also common. With Dior's "New Look", dresses and hats became larger again and if anything, it became more, not less, expected that stylish women would wear hats. The shallow, wide-brimmed saucer-hat was popular at first, giving way to smaller, neater styles. Finally, the signature of Jackie Kennedy – the pillbox – was in vogue during the late 1950s and early 1960s, when fashion relinquished the hat as an essential accessory for women thanks to a combination of more relaxed dress codes and the burgeoning women's liberation movement.

HATS TODAY

Few women wear hats regularly unless they happen to be a member of a royal family or on formal diplomatic business. Leaving aside practical hats for cold weather (a simple cashmere beanie, or fur-trimmed Russian-style is fine), there are occasions when hat wearing is expected. Given that women no longer have to wear them anymore, it is quite nice to be presented with the opportunity to do so.

WEDDINGS

The most common time to wear a hat is at a wedding, but choose appropriately. If you are wearing a classic shift and long coat, a straw hat in the same colour (purists would demand the same fabric, too) with a wide brim and some sort of trim is your safest bet. However, if you like to make a statement there is no reason not to choose a more flamboyant design, so long as the colour matches. Always try a potential hat on with your complete outfit before making a purchase or hiring (hat hire companies are an excellent idea if you rarely have cause to wear one).

If you are wearing a younger, more fashion-forward dress, a "piece" or smaller hat might be more appropriate. Fascinators, as they are known

– mostly feathery affairs attached to a hair comb – can look elegant although they have become somewhat ubiquitous, which detracts from their style somewhat. Source an original one or wear a bejewelled comb or flower.

COCKTAIL HATS
There was a time when women always wore small hats with cocktail dresses. Although the custom is far less common these days, this is an elegant way to smarten up a plain cocktail dress and has a lovely vintage feel about it.

SUMMER HATS
Protecting a delicate complexion from the sun may be essential to maintain ones looks but there is no need for an excuse to wear a lovely straw summer hat. A wide-brimmed, scarf-trimmed straw worn with large sunglasses is inimitably chic and, if you can carry it off, a more masculine-style Panama or fedora is redolent of 1930s Chanel androgyny and looks good with a floaty floral summer dress. Avoid baseball caps at all costs!

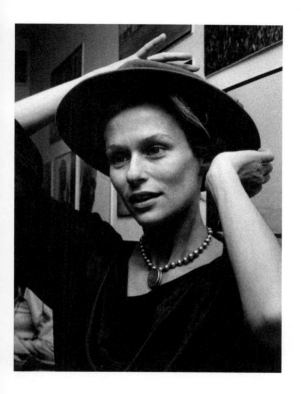

Lauren Hutton, 1975.

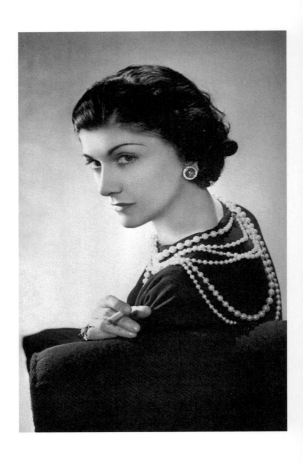

*Coco Chanel made pearls an essential accessory
for the society lady.*

JEWELLERY

THE HISTORY OF JEWELLERY

The human need for adornment is a long-standing one and it is thought that we have been fashioning objects into a kind of jewellery for an incredible 75,000 years – the earliest recorded beads were made of snail shells, and beads created from ostrich egg shells date back 40,000 years. Cro-Magnons, the first Homo sapiens to inhabit Europe 35,000 years ago, made crude jewellery from animal bones (which they sometimes roughly carved), animal teeth and stones, strung to make a necklace or bracelet. In Germany 30,000 years ago, carved mammoth tusks were fashioned into charms. Mother-of-pearl was used early on – ancient Egyptians used pieces in necklaces in 4,000 BC – its incandescent lustre an obvious choice for decoration, and freshwater pearls are mentioned in ancient Chinese texts from 2,000 BC. The first use of copper in jewellery was recorded 7,000 years ago.

As with so many things, it was the ancient Egyptians who are credited with truly establishing the art of jewellery making. Gold was their preferred metal and they admired its rarity and prestige and also appreciated the metal's malleability when it came to crafting. Glass, precious stones and gold were all used to create jewellery worn in life to indicate status and buried with the owner after their death.

Jewellery making also emerged rapidly elsewhere: both the Greeks and Romans used gold and precious stones, including amethysts, pearls and emeralds. The Romans had an extraordinarily diverse toolbox of jewellery-making materials, as wide-ranging as glass beads, bronze, bone and amber and in England a type of fossilized wood was even used. They are credited with the invention of the brooch and produced many ornate versions to hold clothing together. Despite the fall of the Roman Empire, European communities continued to excel in jewellery-making, the Celts being one of the most innovative, achieving an extraordinary quality.

As mentioned, jewellery was worn both for adornment and status but also as a talisman, thought to protect against the Evil Eye. The practice of burying owners with their jewels remained common until the advent of Christianity in the early Middle Ages, hence the wealth of archaeological evidence of jewellery, including necklaces, earrings, combs, buckles, rings and hairpins.

The advance of trade relations during the Renaissance period allowed a further expansion of jewellery-making techniques as cultures learned from one another and were also afforded a greater diversification of gems. Sapphires were imported early on, but emeralds, rubies, turquoise, opals, garnets and amethysts were among many commonly used precious and semi-precious stones. Diamonds, of course, were highly prized and in the 1660s, a merchant named Jean-Baptiste Tavernier imported the stone eventually crafted into the legendary Hope Diamond into France. Diamonds were beloved of the French people, in part thanks to Napoleon Bonaparte, who prized grand jewellery and bedecked both his wives in extravagant sets of diamonds comprised of a matching tiara, earrings, rings, necklace and brooch. Cameos, their images hand-carved from shells or precious stones, were also beloved of Napoleon, just as they were a few decades later by Queen Victoria.

The nineteenth century witnessed a great change in the accessibility of jewellery: the Industrial Revolution brought down the cost of production and also introduced costume jewellery made of paste. At the top end of the market, renowned makers, including Tiffany, Fabergé and Bulgari, all opened their doors during this time. Following the untimely death of her beloved husband Albert in 1861, Queen Victoria introduced mourning jewellery made from black jet, which quickly gained popularity. By the close of the century, Art Nouveau jewellery with its swirls, flourishes and motifs, including animals and flowers had become popular but by the 1920s and '30s, this had given way to the contrasting Art Deco movement, with an emphasis on simple, often-geometric shapes. Manufacturing techniques and the use of new materials has allowed modern jewellery to explore many different fashions, however our love of vintage shows no signs of abating. Some of the most precious and famous jewels in the world sell for extraordinary prices – for example, in the sale of Elizabeth Taylor's jewellery a sixteenth-century pearl necklace fetched $11.8 m (£7.6 m) and the actress's 33.19 carat diamond ring $8.8 m (£5.7 m).

WHAT TO WEAR TODAY

In modern times, the well-dressed lady is fortunate enough to be able to choose between classic jewels and more modern statement pieces. The following all add elegance in different ways.

DIAMONDS

Truly a girl's best friend, a classic diamond ring (even if not an engagement or eternity ring), a single diamond on a fine silver chain (as popularized by Tiffany) or a pair of diamond studs are all suitable for everyday wear. Size might seem important but it is not everything and a discreet diamond has an understated chic about it. For more formal occasions, an Art-Deco diamond brooch, diamond drop earrings or a diamond line bracelet are the height of classic elegance.

PEARLS

Fashionable for centuries, the reputation of pearls as icons of chic was sealed when Coco Chanel accessorized all her outfits with strings and strings of beautiful examples. Today, pearls are universal – always worn by royals but equally coveted by teenage fashion lovers (albeit probably not real ones). A short, single or double rope of pearls is the stalwart of 1950s chic and still worn by many image-conscious, yet classic women today for formal daytime occasions – for example, First Lady Michelle Obama.

For a more fashion-forward look, a longer string of pearls is often teamed with a white shirt, plus a jacket and even smart jeans, or worn for evening on a plain black cocktail dress. Taking their cue from icons of the past including Audrey Hepburn and Elizabeth Taylor, well-dressed women of all ages – among them Sarah Jessica Parker, Angelina Jolie and Oprah Winfrey – all wear pearls regularly.

COSTUME JEWELLERY

Though invented in the eighteenth century, costume jewellery was at its most popular in the twentieth century during the Art Deco period, when it was introduced by Coco Chanel to complete an outfit. Made from imitation gemstones and inexpensive metals such as pewter or nickel, it was once considered inferior to real jewellery but has lately become extremely fashionable and collectable, with some vintage costume jewellery now fetching as much as real diamonds. Stylish women who have worn costume jewellery include Jackie Kennedy and Princess Diana. And there is no reason why the modern well-dressed lady should not wear high-quality costume jewellery because it can be more affordable and just as elegant.

MODERN JEWELLERY

Today, jewellery making is as vibrant as ever, with some wonderful, original pieces being produced. It is worth seeking out modern jewellers to invest in statement necklaces, interesting rings or bold cuffs to accessorize simple, chic outfits.

HANDBAGS

A HISTORY OF HANDBAGS

Small bags, pouches and purses – precursors to the handbags of today – have been around for as long as people had precious items to carry in them. ancient Egyptian hieroglyphics depict men with pouches fastened to the waist and in the Bible Judas Iscariot is described as the "purse carrier", meaning he was the money-keeper for the Apostles. By the fourteenth century, both sexes began to wear girdles – a type of belt with a long piece hanging down at the front, which might be plain leather or for the rich, adorned with jewels – to which they attached not only their pouches carrying coins and small valuables but many other items, including girdle books (small books tied to the belt or girdle that could be swung upwards and easily read), rosaries, keys and fragrant scented pomanders to combat the poor hygiene of the day. While some purses were plain, many women already favoured ornate drawstring versions.

By the Elizabethan era women's fashion was so voluptuous that the tiny medieval girdle pouches would be lost among layer upon layer of skirts. Instead sixteenth-century women began to wear pouches beneath their skirts; again, purses were used for carrying valuables but they also tucked separate small bags full of sweet-smelling herbs such as lavender between layers of clothing (particularly in the case of aristocratic women) to distract from the continued problem of bad smells due to lack of public and personal hygiene. Peasants and travellers began to wear satchel-like leather or rough cloth bags slung diagonally across their body, but higher classes refused obvious bags and throughout the seventeenth century, embroidered purses became more sophisticated, gradually evolving from simple drawstring pouches to more complex shapes and materials.

After the backlash against the aristocracy that followed the French Revolution of 1789–95, women's fashion similarly changed to a simpler silhouette. The voluptuous, ostentatious gowns of Marie Antoinette's day were replaced by unstructured, plain dresses under which there was no space for the loose purses (or "pockets", as they were often called). Instead "reticules" appeared – delicate pouches, usually drawstring, made from a wide variety of materials and adorned with brocade, beading or embroidery. By now women were completely reliant on the small everyday items they carried with them, leading the English to label these early handbags "indispensables".

It was in the mid-nineteenth century that the term "handbag" came into popular usage. This was the era of the railroad and with increased numbers of both men and women travelling regularly, capacious luggage became essential. Until now purses had been fashioned by dressmakers or embroidered by the women themselves but with the need for larger, sturdier hand-held bags, professional luggage makers set up business. Many of these, such as Hermès, had previously been saddle-makers and now turned their hand from horse-travel to the needs of railway travellers. In 1837, Hermès bags first came into existence and in 1854, Louis Vuitton began to produce luggage for rich Parisians, including revolutionary flat-bottomed trunks that could be stacked with ease for long-distance travel. It is interesting to note that even today many modern handbags hark back to this early luggage, with locks, keys, frames, pockets and fastenings.

At the turn of the twentieth century the variety of handbags grew enormously. Small drawstring reticules remained popular but structured leather bags, both small with attached necessities like fans or opera glasses, and larger shoulder bags, were also used. In the 1920s and the Jazz Age, beaded clutches became fashionable and for simpler outfits, matching shoes and handbags were the norm. By the 1930s, the styles of handbag still popular today were in use: the classic structured handbag with its rigid frame, clasp and short handles, the shoulder bag, the satchel and the clutch were all popular and often influenced by the Art Deco movement with abstract designs.

During the Second World War, a more utilitarian shoulder bag influenced by military style was used (by necessity larger as it had to carry items such as gas masks). In the 1950s, however, glamour reigned once more and the cult of the designer handbag was born. Handbags by Chanel and Hermès were colour coordinated with outfits, including shoes and hats, and to complement Christian Dior's New Look, women carried an exaggeratedly feminine tiny handbag. In the 1960s and '70s, handbags continued to follow fashions and everything from small chain-strapped shoulder bags to large satchels and ethnic fabric bags appeared. By the 1980s and '90s, conspicuous consumption and label-mania led to a further rise in the popularity of blatant, logo-heavy designer handbags, along with many fakes. Unisex bags, often in utilitarian fabrics such as black nylon, also became fashionable, although designer labels such as the Prada silver triangle were still important.

Over the last decade the cult of the handbag has reached epidemic proportions, with many fashion-conscious women expecting to buy a new one each season. The cost has also become extraordinarily high, with waiting lists and celebritiy endorsements heralding the latest must-have version.

ESSENTIAL HANDBAG STYLES

CLASSIC HERMÈS-STYLE KELLY

For many women, particularly those who aspire to elegant, classic European style, the Hermès bag is the holy grail of handbags. Iconic designs, including the "Kelly" (named for Grace Kelly) and the "Birkin" (for Jane Birkin) are beautifully crafted, hand-held bags with simple straps and a lock clasp. Capacious, comfortable to carry and instantly recognizable, they are both practical and stylish. Fortunately this style of bag has been much copied and if you can source a similar design in good-quality leather, there is no need to spend so much.

If buying a label is important to you, choose a classic brand that will stand the test of time. Most designers now produce their own beautiful bags, many with an instant recognition factor, but a tradition of quality and craftsmanship should always be of the highest importance. Investment brands with mileage include Mulberry, Bottega Veneta, Yves Saint Laurent and Céline. Neutral colours are most useful although a statement bag in red or Hermès orange is tempting.

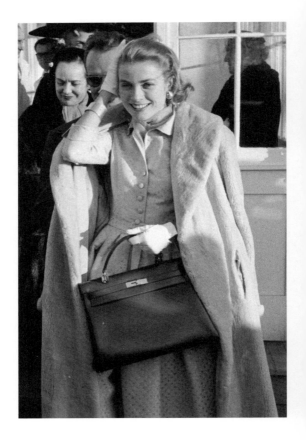

Grace Kelly with the Hermès Kelly bag.

SATCHEL OR SADDLE BAG

While the tote is the most practical and classic day bag, particularly for working women who need to carry laptops, iPads, paperwork and spare heels, the cross-body satchel has recently become extremely popular and has a slightly younger, more casual and contemporary feel. The best satchels are reasonably sized and can also be carried in the hand. A simple, beautifully crafted glossy leather saddle bag is another smart alternative for off-duty days.

SHOULDER BAG

Classic as it comes, every well-dressed woman should own at least one shoulder bag. Again, a simple design and the highest-quality leather are essential. Bottega Veneta's woven *intrecciato* designs are some of the most covetable.

THE TOTE/SHOPPER

An essential item for carrying groceries and shopping, this deep rectangular bag will pull together your look and is a million light years from the plastic carrier bag. Foldable versions, such as those by Longchamps, can be placed in a shoulder bag when not in use.

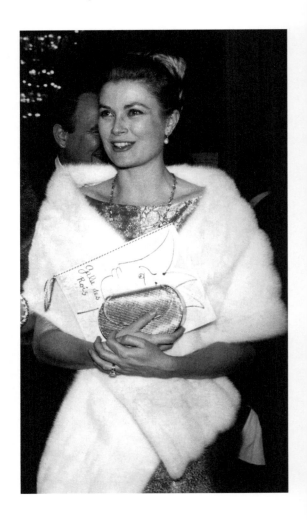

EVENING BAG

Every woman needs a smart evening bag, either a clutch or a simple, thin-strapped shoulder bag. This should be small and have some kind of detail. Although it is usually best to err on the side of simplicity for evening, particularly if your outfit is classic, a bejewelled, gilt-strapped bag can make an elegant statement. Another chic option is to carry a vintage evening bag or purse.

YOUR WARDROBE

CREATING A CAPSULE WARDROBE

Most women have far too many clothes and if you believe, as every well-dressed woman should, that quality is more important than quantity, paring your existing garments down into a capsule collection is essential. Once you have built up a core wardrobe you can invest in one or two extra key pieces that will pull together the items you already possess, allowing you to easily create subtly different outfits and stay classic but never out-of-date instead of buying a "new wardrobe" each season.

Women who aspire to classic, elegant style should take note that all apparently effortlessly chic females have a formula for what they wear. Take Jackie Kennedy, for example: her formal daywear comprised of a shift dress (worn alone or with a jacket) or a skirt suit, with matching shoes, gloves and pillbox hat, accessorized with pearls, sometimes a headscarf and oversized sunglasses.

Her off-duty look tended more towards tailored trousers or neat pencil skirts and simple knitwear such as polo-necks or twinsets; eveningwear consisted of elegant gowns and statement jewellery. Within this framework she was able to play with bright colours, fashionable prints and changing fashions (for example, flared trouser suits towards the 1970s) without losing her own style identity. The former First Lady rightly remains one of our most notable twentieth-century style icons and a modern version of her template will always stand you in good stead, style-wise.

Once you have identified your shape and silhouette (*see pages* 10–7), consider your lifestyle and the style most appropriate to you as an individual by answering the following questions: What age are you? Do you work in a smart office or are you based from home? Are you a professional or a stay-at-home mother? And what is your budget?

Practical issues need to be looked at, too, although practicality does not preclude style. If you have to walk everywhere, high heels may not be suitable but luckily, ballet flats are just as stylish, and should you find yourself treading on the backs of long, wide trousers and ripping the hems, no matter how much you like the look, choose narrow ones. Ask yourself if you can afford to dry clean everything – for example, smart dresses tend to need dry cleaning after each wear whereas a simple top beneath a jacket and skirt can be machine-washed at home.

ESSENTIAL PIECES

The minimum capsule wardrobe consists of the following pieces:

Two pairs of trousers: Choose two smart pairs or one smart and one more casual; wide-legged or narrow tailored according to your shape, in fabrics such as wool or cotton twill and in neutral colours – perhaps one dark, one light. You might like to add a further pair of cropped Capri pants for summer.

One pair of smart jeans: A good fit is essential, so choose skinny leg or bootcut as appropriate; dark denim is most flattering.

Two skirts: A classic pencil or A-line skirt is best, again according to shape. If you suit both, opt for a neutral, plain pencil skirt and a printed silk A-line skirt that can double as eveningwear.

One dress: The most classically elegant and versatile style is the shift dress.

Two plain blouses or shirts: A silk blouse is always chic, as is a crisp white shirt.

Two simple tops or knitted sweaters: Plain round- or polo-neck fine knits (in cashmere or merino wool) are best and will pair well with either skirts or trousers. A twinset or simple neat cardigan could be another option and for Spring/Aummer, a further addition is a well-fitting, boat-neck, striped Breton top.

A good jacket: The most versatile and useful is a blazer-style that goes as well with jeans as smarter trousers. You may need to wear a suit to work, in which case keep that jacket as part of the suit, but consider buying both trousers and skirt or shift dress to match.

Trench coat: An effortless way to look well dressed and practical for spring showers, too. It also goes with everything, instantly giving your outfit some Parisian chic, especially when accessorized with a silk scarf and, if appropriate, sunglasses.

Winter coat: According to your taste, shape and style, a neutral, well-made winter coat is essential. A princess or topcoat style will work for most looks. Investing in quality is always worthwhile.

One evening dress: Either a classic Little Black Dress (LBD) that may be accessorized to give different looks or, if you crave making an entrance on occasion, a stunning evening dress, for example in a statement colour, or classic black but embellished with beads or Swarovski-style glittering crystals.

Shoes: One pair of flats – ballet flats, loafers or driving shoes according to taste and style. One pair of heels – kitten, high stilettos or simple courts (again, consider lifestyle and taste); plus one pair of sandals.

Bags: One large day bag (a classic tote is most practical) and one small evening bag, perhaps beaded and/or vintage.

Accessories: When you work with a capsule wardrobe, accessories are the best way to seasonally update your clothes and create different outfits. Scarves are an instant transformation, both classic silk squares and more modern printed chiffon styles; simple jewellery ensures daytime elegance while a few pieces of statement jewellery for formal and eveningwear are a good investment. A pair of Jackie Kennedy style oversized sunglasses is also inimitably chic.

WARDROBE MAINTENANCE

If you want to build a classic wardrobe that will last you for years, then investing in good-quality garments is only the first step. Caring for those clothes so you get the most wear out of them and to ensure they do not look prematurely shabby is also essential.

STORAGE

Clothes should be stored seasonally; clean and pack away obviously weather-appropriate items such as heavy knits and summer dresses in sealed bags at the end of each season. There are fantastic vacuum bags you can buy (suck the air out of them with a domestic vacuum cleaner so that they become virtually flat, making space saving easy). Large items such as coats should always be hung on wooden hangers, dry cleaned at the end of each season and left in the cleaner's bag to protect from dust, moths or accidental damage. Dry cleaning also kills any moth eggs lurking about. In general, the odour of cedar balls will repel moths, but only cleaning to remove eggs and packing in an airtight bag afterwards will ensure no moth holes.

The clothes you wear regularly should be stored in a wardrobe with enough space between each item. Fold knitwear and casual tops; place everything else on wooden hangers. Periodically clear out your sock and underwear drawer – if you are feeling self-indulgent, discard and replace the lot! Bras should ideally be replaced every six months.

SHOE AND STORAGE BAGS

Store smart shoes with wooden shoehorns inside; boot-trees are essential for high boots. If space is not an issue, keeping shoes in their original boxes is a good idea, or at least in shoe bags on a shoe rack. Shoes are particularly susceptible to dampness and mildew, as are leather handbags – stuffing bags with crumpled paper and leaving them unfastened will help prevent this. They also need to be wiped with a cloth every so often to prevent mildew from building up around the soles (keep in boxes if the problem is bad). Store handbags in a soft drawstring cotton bag.

Leather and suede shoes and bags should always be sprayed with a protective spray before use and intermittently afterwards. Polish your shoes regularly and wipe over handbags with a fine cloth. If made from hard leather (for example, a saddle bag), polish with beeswax-based leather cream.

WASHING

Knitwear should really be handwashed or dry cleaned. Some pieces will be fine on a cool wool-cycle of your washing machine (in my experience, cashmere is more resilient than fine merino wool). Clothing labels usually advise handwashing regardless. Silk should be handwashed or washed in the delicates cycle of your machine. Cotton has a tendency to shrink, so wash on a cooler rather than super-hot cycle (it also fades quickly when washed too often). Formal dresses, skirts, jacket and coats all require regular dry cleaning.

ALTERING

Lastly it is worth remembering that clothes can be altered, if necessary – either when first bought to ensure a flawless fit, or if your figure changes over the years, or even to bring an item in line with fashion. It is almost unheard of today but, for generations, women had skirts taken up according to trends, items let out and shoulder pads made larger or smaller according to that season's silhouette. There is much to be said for a sustainable wardrobe that lasts years rather than the disposable attitude of discarding cheap clothes after just a few wears. And never worry about recycling your outfits – the Duchess of Cambridge has made this perfectly acceptable.

ACKNOWLEDGEMENTS

The publishers would like to thank the following
sources for their kind permission to reproduce the
pictures in this book.

Key: t=Top, b=Bottom, c=Centre, l=Left and r=Right

Image Courtesy of The Advertising Archives: 97,
145

Getty Images: /Gamma-Keystone: 34, 146, /Gamma-
Rapho: 66, /Hulton Archive: 84, 91, 128, 136, 158, /
Mondadori: 93, /Time & Life Pictures: 4, 18, 180, 180,
/Roger Viollet: 166, /WireImage: 165

Mary Evans Picture Library: 8, /Illustrated London
News: 111, /National Magazine Company: 38

Rex Features: /ADC: 30, /Europress: 182, /Everett
Collection: 54

Every effort has been made to acknowledge correctly
and contact the source and/or copyright holder of
each picture and Carlton Books Limited apologizes for
any unintentional errors or omissions, which will be,
corrected in future editions of this book.